Case Presentations in (Medicine

Other titles published

Case Presentations in Renal Medicine
Case Presentations in Paediatrics
Case Presentations in Cardiology
Case Presentations in Gastrointestinal Disease
Case Presentations in General Surgery

In preparation

Case Presentations in Urology

Case Presentations in Clinical Geriatric Medicine

G. S. Rai, MD, MSc, MRCP
Consultant Physician in Geriatric Medicine, Whittington and Royal Northern Hospitals, and
Senior Lecturer, University College Hospital Medical School, London

P. J. Murphy, MB, MRCPI
Senior Research Fellow and Locum Consultant Physician, Whittington and Royal Northern Hospitals, London

G. Wright, MB, BSc, MRCP
Clinical Lecturer and Honorary Senior Registrar, Whittington Hospital, London

Butterworths
London Boston Durban Singapore Sydney Toronto Wellington

First published, 1987

British Library Cataloguing in Publication Data

Rai, G. S.
Case presentations in clinical geriatric medicine
–(case presentations)
1. Geriatrics–Diseases–Diagnosis–Case studies
I. Title II. Murphy, P. J. III. Wright, G.
618.97'075 RC953

ISBN 0-407-01480-2

Phototypesetting by En to En, Tunbridge Wells
Printed and bound in Great Britain by Anchor Brendon Ltd, Tiptree, Essex

Preface

The practice of geriatric medicine differs in many respects from that of young adult medicine. In the elderly, diseases are more likely to present atypically, history is sometimes unavailable and physical signs are often non-specific or even absent altogether. Multiple pathologies frequently coexist and the elderly are much more vulnerable to environmental and iatrogenic insults. In addition, physical problems are sometimes overshadowed by social problems in the elderly and the team approach is of paramount importance.

We have tried to illustrate some of these differences by using cases based on patients who have been referred to us and treated by the Department of Geriatric Medicine. Consequently some of the cases are very 'grey' and in some the management may be open to question.

As a specialty, geriatric medicine is now included in the examination for the diploma of MRCP(UK) by the Royal Colleges of Physicians. In addition, the Royal College of Physicians of London has set up a new examination for the Diploma in Geriatric Medicine. This is designed for general practitioner's vocational trainees, clinical assistants and other doctors working in non-consultant career posts in departments of geriatric medicine. Both these examinations have clinical sections consisting of long and short cases.

Although this book is not a comprehensive guide to the specialty of geriatric medicine, it should prove useful to those qualified physicians preparing for both types of diploma examinations. Other physicians who deal with the elderly and final year medical students should also find it useful and stimulating, for it clearly demonstrates that geriatric medicine does not just comprise strokes, arthritis and senile dementia.

G. S. Rai
P. J. Murphy
G. Wright

Contents

Part 1

Case Presentations and Questions

Case 1

A 71-year-old woman who lived with an 84-year-old physically disabled husband was referred because of a 3-month history of non-specific illness associated with abnormal liver function tests. On direct questioning the only symptom she admitted to having was neck pain. On examination, she had reduced neck movements and facet joint tenderness.

Investigations

Haemoglobin: 12.4 g/dl
ESR: 28 mm in the first hour
SGOT: marginally raised
Hepatitis surface antigen: positive
Auto-antibody screen: negative
Alkaline phosphatase: raised
Gamma GT: raised

X-ray of cervical spine: extensive degenerative changes
Ultrasound of liver and gallbladder: cholelithiasis

Without any specific treatment (apart from local heat treatment to the neck) her liver function tests returned to normal and her neck pain improved. She was therefore discharged from hospital with a follow-up appointment. Three weeks later she returned to the out-patient department complaining of bitemporal headaches, generalized aches and pains, fever of 100–101°F, night sweats, temporomandibular claudication and increased neck pain. There were however, no visual symptoms or scalp tenderness; her ESR at this time was 36 mm in the first hour.

Questions

1. What is the likely cause of her symptoms and how would you confirm the diagnosis?
2. Is the ESR of 36 mm in the first hour compatible with the diagnosis made by you?
3. Could the abnormal liver function tests during her initial admission be explained by the diagnosis made by you in (1)?
4. Name four atypical presentations of this condition?
5. What is the problem that would require the services of a social worker on admission of the patient?

Case 2

A woman of 78 years of age who lived alone was referred with symptoms of a chest infection. During admission she also admitted to having diarrhoea for 6 weeks, weight loss of 1 stone over 6 months and impaired vision in the left eye since childhood. Prior to this admission, i.e. six years earlier she stated that she was diagnosed as having ? colitis and put on sulphasalazine with good effect at another hospital.

On examination, she had a firm tender mass 8 cm in diameter in the left iliac fossa, a regular pulse of 112 beats per minute with an occasional ectopic beat, and a blood pressure of 180/100 mmHg.

Investigations

Haemoglobin: 10.8 g/dl
MCV: 84 fl
Serum iron: 4 μmol/l
TIBC: 48 μmol/l

Albumin: 34 g/l
Alkaline phosphatase: 114 IU/l
AST: 42 IU/l

Amylase: 210 IU/l

Calcium: 2.04 mmol/l
Gamma GT: 45 IU/l
Potassium: 3.2 mmol/l
Sodium: 127 mmol/l
Urea: 3.8 mmol/l

Barium enema: showed long segment of sigmoid colon with abnormal mucosal pattern. The mucosa appeared oedematous and the barium extended between the oedematous folds (resembling cobblestones).

Questions

1. What is the probable diagnosis in this patient?
2. How would you confirm it?
3. What is the management of this condition?

Case 3

A woman of 83 years of age who lived alone with long-standing rheumatoid arthritis (since 1944) was admitted following a fall. At the time of her admission she was pyrexic, had cellulitis of both legs, a painful left knee, widespread changes of rheumatoid arthritis with nodules, in addition to a mass in the left hypochondrium.

Investigations

(a) **Initial investigations**
Haemoglobin: 6.8 g/dl (but 12.3 g/dl after transfusion)
WCC: 3.7×10^9/l (differential showing neutrophil count of 53%)
Platelets: 364×10^9/l (with blood film being diamorphic)

(b) **One month later**
Haemoglobin: 10.1 g/dl
WCC: 2.8×10^9/l
Platelet count: 246×10^9/l
Serum iron: 2.5 μmol/l
TIBC: 54 μmol/l
T4: 79 nmol/l

Barium meal: showed only hiatus hernia.
Liver scan: showed patchy uptake of ^{99m}TC sulphur colloid, and increased uptake by an enlarged spleen.

Questions

1. What are the diagnoses in this woman?
2. What is the cause of the liver scan appearance?
3. What will be the management of this patient?

Case 4

A 92-year-old woman living in Part III accommodation was referred to the day hospital because of immobility due to pain in the right knee. On examination she had an inflamed swelling of the right knee with clinical evidence of an effusion.

Investigations

Haemoglobin: 11.9 g/dl
WCC: 8.1×10^9/l

Albumin: 36 g/l
Alkaline phosphatase: 74 IU/l
AST: 11 IU/l
Bilirubin: 24 mmol/l
Calcium: 2.32 mmol/l
Glucose: 6 mmol/l
Phosphate: 0.89 mmol/l
Urate: 0.2 mmol/l

X-ray of right knee showed changes of osteoarthritis with calcification of articular cartilages.

Questions

1. What is the diagnosis and how would you confirm it?
2. Name 4 well-known associations of this condition?
3. How would you treat this patient?
4. What is the cause of raised bilirubin?

Case 5

An 81-year-old man was admitted to hospital following a syncopal attack. He described this as 'an episode of faintness' followed by collapse and loss of consciousness. There was no history of tongue biting, incontinence or headache. He had approximately seven similar episodes over the previous 20 years. Following one of these a 24 hour ECG tape showed SVT which was treated with digoxin.

Clinical examination revealed a heart rate of 80 beats/min with an occasional ectopic beat, blood pressure of 120/60 mmHg (supine) and 100/50 mmHg (erect). CNS examination was otherwise normal.

Questions

1. What further details should be elicited from the history?
2. What simple bedside test might yield valuable information?
3. How should syncopal attacks be investigated?
4. What is the treatment for postural hypotension?

Case 6

A 70-year-old right-handed man was admitted having 'gone off his feet' following a fall during an alcoholic binge some days before. He was a known alcoholic but was taking no medication. Past medical history included diabetes mellitus controlled with diet, peptic ulceration confirmed by barium meal and a head injury in 1977 when he also sustained a fracture of cervical vertebrae and needed to be in hospital for traction.

On examination he was dry and apyrexial. He was confused and disorientated in time. There was a bruise on the left side of his forehead. His pulse was a regular 80 beats/min with a blood pressure of 155/90 mmHg. Heart sounds were audible and he had a soft ejection systolic murmur heard in the aortic area. No abnormalities were detected in the chest or abdomen and there were no focal neurological signs.

Investigations

Haemoglobin: 14.8 g/dl
WCC: $7.8 \times 10^9/l$
Platelets: $350 \times 10^9/l$

Glucose: 6.2 mmol/l
Potassium: 4.2 mmol/l
Sodium: 137 mmol/l
Urea: 9.5 mmol/l

Skull X-rays: normal
EEG: evidence of midline disturbance and marked asymmetry
CT scan: superficial, subdural low-density mass over the right frontoparietal region with marked mass effect.

Questions

1. What is the cause of this man's confusion?
2. What are the possible aetiological factors of this condition in this patient?
3. Is confusion a typical way of presentation of this condition?

Case 7

A 77-year-old spinster who lived in a warden controlled flat with home help once a week, was admitted with a several month history of epigastric and retrosternal discomfort on eating and a 1-week history of lethargy and anorexia. On direct questioning, she admitted to having passed orange-coloured urine for the last few months, although she was unaware that she was jaundiced. In the past, she had a colectomy for ulcerative colitis 24 years earlier. For the past several months she had taken diclofenac.

On examination she was jaundiced but there was no evidence of itching. Although her palms were red there were no other cutaneous features of acute or chronic liver disease. Her pulse was 80 beats/min regular, blood pressure 120/80 mmHg and in the abdomen she had a smooth but tender liver 2 cm below the costal margin.

Investigations

Haemoglobin: 13.9 g/dl
WCC: 8.4×10^9/l
Platelet count: normal

AST: 1030 IU/l
Alkaline phosphatase: 333 IU/l
Bilirubin: 155 μmol/l
Random blood glucose: 8.8 mmol/l

Hepatitis B antigen: negative
Smooth muscle antibody: strongly positive
Clotting times: normal
Chest X-ray: revealed calcification in both lung fields, particularly the apices where there was fibrotic change.
Liver ultrasound: revealed the common bile duct to be at the upper limit of normal with no intra-hepatic biliary tract dilatation, also a solitary stone was noticed in the gall bladder.

Questions

1. What diagnoses would you make in this woman and how would you confirm this?
2. What will be your management of jaundice in this patient?

Case 8

A woman of 82 years of age who lived alone in a third floor flat and was receiving home help twice weekly and meals-on-wheels five days a week, was admitted with a 2-month history of pruritus associated with jaundice. There was no history of heavy alcohol ingestion but the patient had been on prochlorperazine. On direct questioning she admitted to having pale stools and dark urine over the previous 2 weeks.

On examination she was deeply jaundiced with scratch marks and a vague mass was just palpable on deep palpation in the right hypochondrium.

Investigations

Haemoglobin: 11.8 g/dl
MCV: 87 fl
WCC: 3.2×10^9/l
Prothrombin time: 14 s
PTTK: 35 s

AST: 116 IU/l
Albumin: 36 g/l
Alkaline phosphatase: 690 IU/l
Bilirubin: 22.1 mmol/l
Calcium: 2.19 mmol/l
Glucose: 5.9 mmol/l
Potassium: 3.6 mmol/l
Phosphate: 1.09 mmol/l
Sodium: 134 mmol/l
Urea: 4.9 mmol/l

Questions

1. What is the differential diagnosis?
2. How would you manage this patient?

Case 9

A 67-year-old man, an ex-cigarette smoker, presented to his general practitioner with malaise, weight loss and lethargy. He was found to have clinical signs of consolidation in his left upper lobe and was therefore treated with courses of ampicillin and cotrimoxazole. Since this therapy had no beneficial effect he was referred to hospital for admission.

Clinical examination and chest X-rays confirmed the consolidation in the left upper lobe. In addition, he was confused but there was no other clinical abnormality. Two days after admission he had a normal bronchoscopic examination including bronchial brushings and biopsy.

Investigations

Normal except for an ESR of 79 mm in the first hour.

Questions

1. What are the most likely diagnostic possibilities?
2. What investigations should be done?
3. How should he be treated?
4. What are the possible causes for his confusion?

Case 10

An 89-year-old woman was referred to hospital with dizziness. There was no history of chest pain, palpitations or vertigo. There was, however, a long history of diarrhoea and abdominal distension including an urticarial skin rash associated with swelling of her left eyelid, the left side of her face, tongue and lips. The urticarial rash was intermittent and had been occurring over a 6-month period. She denied having any stridor or dysphagia.

On examination, the positive findings were local weals and erythema over the arm, trunk, lips, right ear, and also a distended abdomen. An abdominal X-ray revealed gaseous distension of the sigmoid colon.

Questions

1. List 4 causes of urticaria?
2. Is the skin rash related to the abdominal symptoms?
3. What laboratory tests would you carry out for the urticarial rash?
4. What is the treatment of this condition?

Case 11

An 89-year-old West Indian man who lived alone and had been confined to his flat for 6 months, was admitted after a 2-month history of increasing back pain. There was no history of trauma or weakness. In the past he had had a partial gastrectomy for peptic ulceration many years earlier.

On examination the positive findings were swollen metacarpal phalangeal joints, ulnar deviation of fingers, tenderness to percussion over the lumbar spine and bowing of both tibiae.

Investigations

Haemoglobin: 13.5 g/dl
MCV: 94 fl
WCC: 4.0×10^9/l

Acid phosphatase: 2.6 IU/l
Albumin: 44 g/l
Alkaline phosphatase: 206 IU/l
AST: 41 IU/l
Calcium: 2.17 mmol/l
Glucose: 4.7 mmol/l
Phosphate: 1.22 mmol/l

ESR: 6 mm in first hour
ECG: showed flutter or fibrillation
X-ray of hands: erosion of base of proximal phalanx of fourth finger on the left side and at distal radio-ulnar joints
X-ray of pelvis: irregular patches of increased density present with coarsened trabecular pattern
X-ray of lumbosacral spine: coarse trabeculation with cortical thickening
larger vertebrae than thoracic vertebrae
narrowing of intervertebral disc spaces with osteophytes and spondylolisthesis of L4 and L5.

Questions

1. What is(are) the factor(s) responsible for the back pain?
2. What are the complications of the bone disease present in this man?
3. What treatment would you give to the patient?

Case 12

A 94-year-old woman was admitted with 2-week history of dyspnoea and productive cough. On direct questioning she denied having any paroxysmal nocturnal dyspnoea, chest pain or palpitations, but admitted to experiencing wheezing particularly in the mornings over the preceding 3 years.

On examination the only abnormal sign she had was an expiratory wheeze audible through both lung fields.

Investigations

Haemoglobin: 14.1 g/dl
WCC: 7.0×10^9/l (73% neutrophils, 15% lymphocytes, 1% monocytes)
Chest X-ray: normal
ECG: T-wave changes in lateral leads
Peak expiratory flow rate: 55 l/min.

Questions

1. What is the diagnosis?
2. What are other clinical features of acute attack of this condition which were not present in this patient?
3. What problems would you envisage with therapy on discharge?

Case 13

An 86-year-old widow who lived alone was having increasing difficulty in coping with life. She had become increasingly confused over a 2-year period and had fallen several times prior to admission. She had been incontinent of urine for a long time but this problem had become much worse in the 2 weeks prior to admission. She lived in her own 3 storey house and 2 nieces visited her regularly. She refused to let anyone else into the house. She had no past medical history and was not taking any regular medication.

Examination revealed a frail elderly lady with a score on the Royal College of Physicians mental test of 4/10. There were no focal neurological signs and the remainder of the examination was completely normal.

Questions

1. What is the diagnosis?
2. What 3 treatable causes of chronic confusion would you be anxious to consider and exclude?
3. What neurobiochemical abnormality has been noted in patients with dementia of Alzheimer type?

Case 14

A 72-year-old man presented to the outpatient clinic with a history of dyspnoea and ankle oedema. He had a past history of hypertension for which he had been taking a thiazide diuretic. There was no family history of either cardiovascular or renal disease.

Clinically he was mildly anaemic. His pulse was 76 beats/min and regular. His blood pressure was 170/90 mmHg and his JVP was raised 4 cm. He had gross peripheral oedema and his apex beat was displaced to the sixth intercostal space in the anterior axillary line. His heart sounds were normal with a grade 3/6 systolic ejection bruit of aortic sclerosis. He had a pericardial friction rub. Examination of his central nervous system was normal and there was no evidence of a peripheral neuropathy or myopathy. His abdomen revealed no bladder or renal enlargement. His prostate gland felt normal on rectal examination.

Investigations

Haemoglobin: 8.6 g/dl
WCC: 5.3×10^9/l

Albumin: 38 g/l
Alkaline phosphatase:

Platelets: $167 \times 10^9/l$

186 IU/l
Bicarbonate: 16 mmol/l
Calcium: 1.89 mmol/l
Potassium: 3.4 mmol/l
Phosphate: 2.6 mmol/l
Sodium: 136 mmol/l
Urea: 64 mmol/l

Questions

1. What is the diagnosis?
2. What other clinical features should one look for on examination that might indicate the aetiology?
3. What are the causes of this condition in the elderly?
4. What is the cause of the pericardial rub?
5. How should this patient be treated?

Case 15

A 90-year-old widow who lived alone in her own house and had not consulted her doctor previously was admitted following a fall. She gave a 6-month history of pain in her thighs and difficulty in climbing stairs. She denied having any illnesses in the past. At the time of admission she was taking phenobarbitone (30 mg) for night sedation and this, according to her, she had taken for the last 30 years.

On examination the positive findings were marked muscle weakness with normal reflexes. Sensation to pin prick and position was also impaired but only at the end of the toes.

Investigations

Haemoglobin: 13.5 g/dl
ESR: 42 mm/l
Liver function: normal
Thyroxine: normal
Urea: normal
Electrolytes: normal

Alkaline phosphatase: 620 IU/l
Calcium: 2.13 mmol/l
Phosphate: 0.77 mmol/l

X-ray of chest: healed fracture of eighth rib present on right side
X-ray of pelvis and femur: no fractures present

Questions

1. What is the cause of this patient's symptoms?
2. How would you confirm the diagnosis?
3. What abnormality would you see on bone scan?
4. What plans would be required before discharge?

Case 16

A 77-year-old woman who lived alone was admitted to our unit via the casualty unit. Three weeks prior to admission she had suffered a 'flu-like' illness and a secondary chest infection resulting in a productive cough. Forty-eight hours before admission she became increasingly short of breath, pyrexial and drowsy. Her drowsiness increased and at the time of admission she was in a comatose state responding to painful stimuli only. Twenty-four hours prior to admission she had been started on erythromycin 500 mg qds by her general practitioner with paracetamol for pain and Benylin for cough.

On examination she was an ill lady in a comatose state. There were no signs of anaemia, jaundice or cyanosis and there was no lymphadenopathy. She had a temperature of 39.9°C, a pulse of 98 beats/min regular and a blood pressure of 160/90 mmHg. The other significant findings were a mid-systolic ejection bruit and scattered rhonchi at both bases. There were no focal neurological signs.

Investigations

Haemoglobin: 13.7 g/dl
WCC: 24.3 × 10^9/l (with predominance of polymorphs—86%)
Platelets: 215 × 10^9/l
ESR: 20 mm in first hour

Liver function: normal
Urea: normal
Glucose: normal
Electrolytes: normal

X-ray of chest: cardiomegaly with mild congestive changes
X-ray of skull: clouding of right mastoid
Lumbar puncture: no rise in pressure but large numbers of polymorphs in the fluid
CSF protein content: 4.06 g/l
CSF glucose: 2.8 mmol/l
Blood glucose: 6.4 mmol/l
Culture of CSF: revealed no growth

Questions

1. What was the cause of her mental impairment?
2. What treatment should she receive?

Case 17

An 87-year-old widow with many years history of increasing confusion was admitted from a home for the elderly with general physical decline associated with anorexia and weight loss. She was disorientated in time and place and denied having any specific symptoms. On examination the only positive finding was the presence of a large left sided pleural effusion.

Investigations

Haemoglobin: 11.5 g/dl
MCV: 80 fl
WCC: $3.7 \times 10^9/l$
Platelet count: $385 \times 10^9/l$
ESR: 40 mm in first hour

Albumin: 33 g/l
Glucose: normal
Urea: normal
Electrolytes: normal:
Liver function tests: normal
Total protein 65 g/l

X-ray of chest: large, left-sided effusion present
Serial sputum examination for AFB: negative
Pleural fluid: straw-colour with the presence of a few lymphocytes but no malignant cells. Protein content of pleural fluid raised
Mantoux tests: 1:10 000 and 1:1000 were negative

Questions

1. What are the likely causes of the pleural effusion?
2. Does negative sputum examination of AFB and negative Mantoux test exclude the presence of tuberculosis in this patient?
3. Would treatment of the effusion improve her physical and mental states?

Case 18

A 73-year-old woman collapsed whilst shopping in a supermarket and was observed to have a grand mal fit. At the time of arrival in casualty the patient was conscious. She had no complaints and no knowledge of the fit.

On examination she had a radial pulse of 60 beats/min which was irregular; however, the apex rate was 160 beats/min with a blood pressure of 90 mmHg systolic. There were no signs of heart failure and no focal neurological signs.

Investigations

(a) **Emergency investigations**
Potassium of 2.7 mmol/l. In view of this she was given 40 mmol/l of KCl over 2 hours and digitalized. On this she reverted to sinus rhythm.

The following day further history from her husband and the patient revealed that: (i) she had been taking Bumetanide-K (1 daily) for oedema of the legs, (ii) had experienced a partial gastrectomy many years ago and (iii) had had frequent, pale stools for the last 3–6 months.

(b) **Further investigations**

Haemoglobin: normal
WCC: normal

Calcium: normal
Phosphate: normal
Serum thyroxine: normal

ECG: normal
3-day faecal fat excretion: 14 mmol/24 hours
^{14}C glycocholic breath test: elevated excretion of $^{14}CO_2$ in her breath within 60 min

Questions

1. What possible aetiological factors produced the hypokalaemia?
2. What ECG changes may have been present at the time of admission apart from atrial fibrillation?
3. What treatment should this patient have on discharge?

Case 19

A 69-year-old woman was admitted with a 10-week history of non-specific malaise, polyuria, polydipsia and, more recently, urinary incontinence.

Examination showed an ill, dehydrated, pigmented woman with Kussmaul's respiration. Her blood pressure was 130/90 mmHg. Abdominal examination was unremarkable apart from massive procidentia.

Investigations

Bicarbonate: 3.4 mmol/l
Potassium: 7.9 mmol/l
Sodium: 128 mmol/l
Urea: 71.5 mmol/l

These values confirmed renal failure.

Questions

1. What is the most likely cause of her renal failure?
2. How much renal function could she expect to recover after treatment?
3. What is the cause of her recent incontinence?

Case 20

A 91-year-old woman who lived alone in a ground floor flat (with support from home help twice weekly, 'meals-on-wheels' 7 days per week and a district nurse) was admitted because of general deterioration. On direct questioning, the patient admitted to having painful itching on the left side of the neck, dyspnoea on slightest exertion and a non-productive cough.

On examination she had a pulse of 98 beats/min in atrial fibrillation and blood pressure of 130/80 mmHg. On the left side, she had excoriations and infected patchy bleeding areas on the ulnar side of upper arm and skin of the axilla. The other abnormal findings were a raised JVP of 4 cm, signs of left pleural effusion and minimal ankle oedema.

Investigations

Haemoglobin: 13.0 g/dl
WCC: 184×10^9/l (with 87% lymphocytes)
Platelet count: 326×10^9/l
Liver function tests: normal

Albumin: normal
Alkaline phosphatase: 357 IU/l
Calcium: normal
Gamma GT: 145 IU/l
Glucose: 5.9 mmol/l
Potassium: normal
Urea: normal
Electrolytes: normal

ECG: atrial fibrillation with T-wave changes in anterolateral leads

X-ray of chest: revealed slightly enlarged heart, marked kyphosis with left pleural effusion and hiatus hernia.

Questions

1. What is the cause(s) of this woman's deterioration?
2. What is the probable cause of her pleural effusion?
3. What complications are likely to be experienced by this woman in the future?

Case 21

An 87-year-old woman with long-standing deforming rheumatoid arthritis (RA) was admitted with pain and swelling of her left shoulder.

Clinical examination revealed a hot, swollen and tender left shoulder joint with clinical evidence of an effusion. Apart from the stigmata of RA, clinical examination was otherwise normal.

Questions

1. What is the differential diagnosis?
2. What essential tests would you do?
3. How should she be treated?
4. What is the prognosis for this condition in the elderly?

Case 22

A woman of 66 years of age presented to hospital following a fall. She gave a 2-month history of increasing difficulty in walking with a tendency to fall. There were no prodromal symptoms to suggest transient ischaemic attacks from cardiac origin or from other vascular pathologies. She had a long history of pain with radiation into the back of her occiput. There was no history of sphincter disturbances. Past medical history included epilepsy since childhood (controlled with phenytoin and phenobarbitone), poor vision in the right eye since 1940 following an accident with a push-bike when she was comatosed for 72 hours, and a patellectomy for osteoarthritis in 1970.

On examination she was a pleasant youthful lady with no anaemia, jaundice or cyanosis. Her pulse was 80 beats/min regular and her blood pressure was 120/90 mmHg. On the short RCP mental test score she scored 10/10, but formal psychometric testing revealed mild intellectual impairment. In addition, she had a right strabismus with a right medial rectus palsy (a long-standing abnormality present since 1940). Fundi and cranial nerves appeared normal on examination. In her musculoskeletal system she had a slight global reduction in power but reflexes were symmetrically exaggerated. Both plantars were flexor. In addition, she had changes of osteoarthritis of the right knee and gravitational ulcers on the left leg.

Investigations

A plain skull X-ray showed abnormalities of the pituitary fossa suggestive of a raised intracranial pressure. A subsequent CT scan revealed marked dilatation of the ventricles with no significant dilatation of the sulci.

Questions

1. What is the likely diagnosis?
2. What is the treatment and the prognosis of this condition?

Case 23

An 85-year-old widow who lived in a ground floor council flat with support from neighbours was admitted with a 4-week history of tiredness, lethargy and dizziness and a 2-week history of polyuria, polydipsia and nocturia. On the day of admission she had fallen resulting in bruising over the right cheek and right supra-orbital region. Her right retina had become detached 10 years earlier, and hypertension had been diagnosed many years before that, for which she was given Moduretic (amiloride and hydrochlorothiazide) in a dose of one tablet daily.

On examination she was alert and orientated. Her pulse was a regular 100 beats/min and her blood pressure 100/80 mmHg lying and 70/40 mmHg standing. No other abnormality was noted on examination.

Investigations

Haemoglobin: 16.1 g/dl
WCC: 9.5×10^9/l
Plasma osmolality: 304 mosm/kg

Calcium: normal
Glucose: 52.5 mmol/l
Potassium: 2.1 mmol/l
Phosphate: normal
Sodium: 117 mmol/l
Thyroxine: normal
Urea: 10.5 mmol/l

Liver function tests: normal
X-ray of chest: normal
ECG: normal
MSU specimen: contained large number of pus cells and culture produced significant growth of *Escherichia coli.*

Questions

1. List the conditions this patient is suffering from?
2. What treatment should this patient receive?

Case 24

A man of 67 years of age was admitted with progressive swelling of his legs. On examination he had a pulse of a regular 84 beats/min, a blood pressure of 150/80 mmHg, normal heart sounds, gross pitting oedema up to and involving the thighs, but normal breath sounds in the chest.

Investigations

Haemoglobin: 16.5 g/dl
WCC: 6.4 × 10^9/l
Prothrombin time ratio: 1.4
Total protein: 59 g/l
Bilirubin: 5 μmol/l

Albumin 27 g/l
Albuminuria: ++++ with 24 h urinary protein excretion of 29 g
Alkaline phosphatase: 129 IU/l
Calcium: 2.10 mmol/l
Potassium: 4.2 mmol/l
SGOT: 19 IU/l
Sodium: 139 mmol/l
Urea: 6.9 mmol/l
Fasting blood glucose: 9.8 mmol/l

α-serum amylase 258 IU/l
α-glycosylated haemoglobin AIC: 8.3%
Creatinine clearance 57 ml/min
Rheumatoid factor: negative
Autoantibody screen: negative

Questions

1. What is the diagnosis (or diagnoses if more than one)?
2. Would renal biopsy be helpful in this patient?
3. How would you treat this patient?

Case 25

A 70-year-old man with long-standing chronic bronchitis was admitted with back pain, intermittent abdominal pain and distension. There was no history of diarrhoea, mucus or blood loss from the gastrointestinal tract. Clinical examination revealed a pulse rate of 85 beats/min, blood pressure of 150/90 mmHg, a very distended abdomen with hyperactive bowel sounds and a reducible inguinal hernia.

Investigations

Haemoglobin: 12.8 g/dl
WCC: $18.3 \times 10^9/l$

Alkaline phosphatase: normal
Calcium: normal
Phosphate: normal
Serum thyroxine: normal
Urea: normal

Abdominal X-ray: dilated loops of bowel
MSU: significant growth of coliform organisms
Flexible sigmoidoscopy: grossly dilated large bowel with no stenosing lesion
Barium enema: confirmed the above findings and revealed no obstructive lesion.

Questions

1. What is the probable diagnosis?
2. Name 4 disorders which can produce this syndrome
3. How should this patient be managed?

Case 26

A man of 76 years of age, a retired coach driver, was admitted with a 2-week history of diarrhoea and repeated falls, shortness of breath and dysgeusia. There was no vomiting and no history of diuretic ingestion. He had had a partial gastrectomy for duodenal ulcer 30 years earlier, peripheral vascular disease for which he required through-knee amputation of the right leg 26 years ago, and carcinoma of the bronchus diagnosed in 1980. Although bronchoscopy and cytology at that time were negative, he was given a course of radiotherapy.

On examination he was alert and not confused, but was deeply pigmented and had generalized muscle wasting. No finger clubbing or lymphadenopathy were present, and breath sounds in the chest were normal. His pulse was a regular 100 beats/min and his blood pressure 160/70 mmHg lying and 150/60 mmHg standing. In the abdomen, the liver was 2 cm below the costal margin with the liver edge being smooth and tender. Examination of the musculoskeletal system revealed generally decreased muscle power in the proximal muscles of all limbs.

Investigations

Haemoglobin: 10 g/dl
ESR: 5 mm in first hour
Urinary osmolality: 366 mmol/l
Plasma osmolality: 294 mmol/l

Glucose: 21 mmol/l
Potassium: 1.5 mmol/l
Sodium: 138 mmol/l
Urea: 10 mmol/l

Arterial blood gases on air: Po_2: 6 kPa
Pco_2: 7.22 kPa
pH: 7.54

Base excess: 19.5 mmol/l
X-ray of chest: revealed right upper lobe shrinkage and ill-defined opacity projected over the first intercostal space on the right.

Questions

1. What is the likely cause of hypokalaemic alkalosis and how would you confirm this?
2. What should be the management of this patient?
3. What would your future plans be for this patient?

Case 27

A 77-year-old woman presented with lethargy, nausea, anorexia and weight loss. Several months earlier she had experienced an episode of vomiting and giddiness and, at that time, a diagnosis of vertebrobasilar ischaemia was made. Her only regular medication was monthly vitamin B12 injection.

On examination she looked unwell. Buccal pigmentation was absent but she had pigmented skin creases (this was not noted 3 months earlier); absent axillary hair; a supine blood pressure of 150/60 mmHg and blood pressure 145/60 mmHg standing. The remainder of the examination was normal.

Investigations

Potassium: 3.9 mmol/l
Sodium: 131 mmol/l

Random glucose: 5.0 mmol/l
Random cortisol: 75 nmol/l
Cortisol 30 min post i.v. injection of 0.25 mg tetracosactrin: 76 nmol/l

Questions

1. What is the probable diagnosis?
2. What importance do you attach to her pigmentation?
3. How would you determine the cause of her low cortisol level?
4. Which drugs can affect the adrenal cortical hormone production?

Case 28

An 83-year-old woman had long-standing depression associated with abdominal pain. For the latter she had had extensive investigations, including laparotomy, but no organic cause had been found for the pain. She had threatened suicide in the past and was admitted as an emergency after having taken an unspecified number of butobarbitone tablets.

Examination revealed a deeply unconscious woman with an absent gag reflex and no response to deep pain. Pupils were equal and reactive; reflexes were bilaterally depressed with equivocal plantar responses. There were no focal neurological signs. She had an irregular pulse with a blood pressure of 110/60 mmHg. She was breathing spontaneously and was not cyanosed.

Questions

1. What would be your immediate management?
2. In the long term how would you manage her depression?

Case 29

A 72-year-old woman with a long-standing history of bone and joint disease was admitted with increasing immobility and back pain without radiation over a 1-year period. For 2 years she had been confined to her flat. There was no history of trauma, weight loss or haemoptysis. She had mild generalized muscle weakness, but no history of diarrhoea, skin rashes or previous abdominal surgery.

Examination was essentially normal apart from evidence of mild obesity and osteoarthritis with limitation of spinal movements.

Investigations

Haemoglobin: 10.3 g/dl
MCV: 74.4 fl
MCH: 24.4 pg
WCC: 9.3×10^9/l
Total protein: 75 g/l
Platelet count: 426×10^9/l
Blood film: revealed anisocytosis and microcytosis

Albumin: 37 g/l
Alkaline phosphatase: 303 IU/l
Calcium: 1.79 mmol/l
Phosphate: 0.75 mmol/l

Barium follow-through revealed flocculation of barium, dilated loops and thickened bowel wall.

Questions

1. What is the diagnosis (or diagnoses)?
2. What further investigations would you perform?
3. How would you treat this patient?

Case 30

A 70-year-old woman was brought to the casualty department by her daughter who said that she had become increasingly drowsy over the previous 3 days. She also gave a 4-week history of occipital headaches. This she described as a heavy pressure which was worse in the evening and when concentrating. Shortly after the onset of headaches, she complained of clumsiness of the left limbs and intermittent 'pins and needles' in the left hand. On the previous day there had been twitching of the left eye and left side of the mouth. In addition her daughter commented on her recent increasing forgetfulness.

On examination she was drowsy but able to answer questions. She was in sinus rhythm with a blood pressure of 170/90 mmHg. Examination of the cardiovascular system, respiratory system and abdomen was unremarkable. Examination of the central nervous system revealed: (i) pupils of equal diameter with normal response to light, (ii) hypertensive changes in the fundi, (iii) left facial asymmetry, (iv) impaired abduction of the left eye, (v) mild weakness of the left arm, (vi) symmetrically brisk reflexes with flexor plantar responses, (vii) astereognosis in the left hand, (viii) impaired joint sense on the left side and (ix) left sensory inattention.

Investigations

Full blood count, urea and electrolytes, blood glucose, ECG and chest X-ray were all normal.

Questions

1. What is the cause of her drowsiness?
2. What is your differential diagnosis?
3. Name one investigation that will be most helpful?

Case 31

A 72-year-old man was admitted with a 1-month history of pain, stiffness and swelling of his hands and legs. A systems review revealed dyspnoea on exertion but no ankle oedema or angina. This patient had a past history of a myocardial infarction and duodenal ulceration. He was presently on no medication. Clinical examination revealed no lymphadenopathy or anaemia, a pulse of 80 beats/min, a blood pressure of 110/60 mmHg with normal heart sounds, bilaterally warm knees with the presence of effusion in the right knee and swollen hands with tethering of skin and a small mouth.

Questions

1. What is the probable diagnosis?
2. What other clinical features would one look for in a patient like this?
3. What other system is commonly involved?
4. How should this condition be managed?

Case 32

A 78-year-old woman, a retired office cleaner, was admitted for investigation of headaches. She had thought that he hypertension for which she was taking bendrofluazide

(5 mg/day) was out of control. After further questioning, it became apparent that the headaches were present mainly on getting out of bed in the mornings and were made worse by straining or coughing.

On examination the positive findings were a regular pulse of 74 beats/min, a blood pressure 200/100 mmHg, marked kyphoscoliosis and slight blurring of disc on fundoscopy in the left eye.

Investigations

Haemoglobin: 10.4 g/dl
WCC: 3.5×10^9/l
ESR: 38 min in first hour

Calcium: normal
Creatinine: 97 μmol/l
Potassium: 3.1 mmol/l
Phosphate: normal
Sodium: 127 mmol/l
Urea: 5.4 mmol/l

Liver function: normal
Protein strip: no abnormality present
Plasma osmolality: 269 mosm/kg
X-ray of skull: showed poorly-defined pituitary fossa
Tomogram of pituitary fossa: showed presence of large intra-sellar mass with enlargement of the sella and thinning of the dorsum sellae.

Questions

1. What type of pituitary pathology is this patient likely to have?
2. What further investigation did she require?
3. What treatment should she receive?

Case 33

An 86-year-old woman, who lived alone in a first floor flat and was supported by her daughter, and a home help twice weekly was admitted after a gradual increasing immobility, anorexia for 3 weeks and faecal and urinary incontinence. In the past she had had a subarachnoid haemorrhage (4 years previously) osteoarthritis and chronic bronchitis. At the time of admission she was taking Multivite Iron tablets, and indomethacin (Indocid). Her daughter also stated that the patient's memory had progressively deteriorated over the last 18 months.

On examination, she was a thin lady with mental test score of 3/10. She had ichthyotic skin. Pulse was 80 beats/min regular, and blood pressure 130/90 mmHg with no evidence of heart failure. The other positive findings were (i) absent pulses below the femoral artery in the right leg, (ii) a regular mobile but firm 1 cm mass in the right breast with inverted nipple, (iii) global diminution of power in muscles and (iv) rectum full of hard faeces.

Investigations

Haemoglobin: 12.7 g/dl
MCV: 85 fl
WCC: 7.8×10^9/l
ESR: 9 mm in first hour

Albumin: 27 g/l
AST: 13 IU/l
Alkaline phosphatase: 110 IU/l
Bilirubin: 8 μmol/l
Calcium: 2.02 mmol/l
Creatinine: 140 μmol/l
Glucose: 7.6 mmol/l
Potassium: 5.2 mmol/l
Phosphate: 0.96 mmol/l
Sodium: 142 mmol/l
Urea: 17.7 mmol/l
Protein: 52 mmol/l

Urine examination: presence of pus cells and significant growth of *E.coli;* on culture
X-ray of chest: normal
X-ray of abdomen: small right kidney and no left kidney demonstrated; also large amount of faeces present in colon and rectum
X-ray of lumbar spine: loss of normal bone density in lumbar vertebrae with disc narrowing at T12, LI and L4/5, with grade I spondylolisthesis at L4/5

ECG: sinus rhythm and presence of changes from old anterior infarction.

Questions

1. What diagnoses would you make in this woman?
2. What initial treatment would you give to this woman for her incontinence?
3. What line of treatment would you take with regard to the breast lump?
4. Would you treat the osteoporosis of spine in this patient?

Case 34

A 71-year-old taxi driver who still worked part-time and had a long history of chronic obstructive airways disease, was admitted with a 2-day history of increasing breathlessness and wheeze followed by an episode on the morning of admission, when he became unresponsive. He had been diagnosed as having chronic renal failure 5 months earlier when an IVU showed bilaterally small kidneys, and signs of the old tuberculosis involving the lymph node in the neck which occurred 25 years earlier could also be seen. He lived with a friend in a second floor flat and, as his friend had been away, he had been eating poorly and had consumed a bottle of vodka in the last 24 hours before admission. He was taking no drugs at the time. This history was obtained from the patient's general practitioner and the patient's family.

On examination his eyes were open, but there was no response to pain. Brain stem reflexes were intact. Pulse was 90 beats/min regular, blood pressure was 130/70 mmHg. Chest was hyper-inflated and there were signs of consolidation at the right base. In the abdomen the liver edge was just palpable. In the central nervous system – reflexes were brisk and the plantars were both up-going.

Investigations

Haemoglobin: 10.6 g/dl
MCV: 97 fl
WCC: 17.3 × 10^9/l
Creatinine: 399 μmol/l
Blood glucose on admission: 0.6 mmol/l
Urea: 22 mmol/l

All other electrolytes: normal
X-ray of chest: revealed patchy shadowing at left lower zone
ECG: showed P pulmonale.

Questions

1. What diagnoses would you make in this patient?
2. What are the probable factors which might have contributed to the production of hypoglycaemia in this patient?
3. What treatment would you give to this patient?

Case 35

A 71-year-old woman was referred with a 1-month history of increasing haematuria, frequency and dysuria but without any loin pain or weight loss. Clinical examination revealed pale mucous membranes, a pulse rate of 72 beats/min, blood pressure 150/90 mmHg with an ejection systolic murmur and stigmata of osteoarthritis.

Investigations

Haemoglobin: 6.8 g/dl
MCV: 76 fl
MCH: 22
WCC: 4.3 × 10^9/l
Urea: 11.1 mmol/l
MSU: frank haematuria

All other examinations, including PR and PV, were normal.

Questions

1. What are the causes of haematuria?
2. How should this patient be investigated?
3. Is ultrasound a good screening test for a renal mass?

Case 36

A 91-year-old woman with a past history of Parkinson's disease, was admitted for rehabilitation following 2 falls. There was no dizziness or loss of consciousness although, on 1 occasion, she had fallen while turning around. Following her falls she developed a productive cough. At the time of visit she was taking Sinemet 110 ½ tablet bd, benzhexol (Artane) 1 mg daily, mefenamic acid 500 mg tds.

On examination, she had lateral entropion in the right eye, dense cataract on the left, cogwheel rigidity in all limbs, coarse crepitations at both bases, fixed flexion deformity of left hip, and bilateral valgus deformity of both knees.

Investigations

Haemoglobin: 12·9 g/dl
WCC: 8×10^9/l
ESR: 40 mm in first hour
MSU: mixed growth on two occasions
Blood culture: sterile

Alkaline phosphatase: 135 IU/l
AST: normal
Bilirubin: normal
Calcium: 2.12 mmol/l
Random glucose: 6.8 mmol/l
Phosphate: 0.6 mmol/l
Electrolytes: normal

X-ray of chest: cardiomegaly with reticular shadowing in both lung fields
ECG: atrial tachycardia with a 3:1 block

Questions

1. What are the probable factors that may have played a part in her falls?
2. What are the long-term complications of Parkinson's disease?
3. What alteration would you make to the anti-Parkinsonian therapy?

Case 37

A 75-year-old woman living with her husband had taken to bed because of painful soles. In the past she had fractured her right femur (which was treated surgically) and had also undergone an appendicectomy.

On examination she was afebrile, had a pulse of 82 beats/min regular and a blood pressure of 145/80 mmHg. The other positive findings were: (i) palpable smooth liver edge 3 finger breadths below the costal margin, (ii) reduced power in all leg muscle groups but with equal tone, (iii) absent reflexes in lower limbs and (iv) reduced sensation to pin-prick, temperature, light touch and vibration in distal limbs. In the legs the loss was up to the mid-thigh in the right leg and to the mid-calf on the left side.

Investigations

MCV 101 fl
ESR: normal
Full blood count: normal
Hbs Ag negative

Albumin: normal
Alkaline phosphatase: 140 IU/l
Bilirubin: normal
Calcium: normal
Gamma GT: 207 IU/l
Globulin: normal
Potassium: 3.1 mmol/l
Phosphate: normal
Random blood sugar: normal
Sodium: 123 mmol/l
Vitamin B12: normal
Folic acid: normal

Chest X-ray: revealed old, calcified opacities at right apex of lung
Liver scan: revealed patchy uptake by liver with increased uptake by spleen and bone marrow.

Questions

1. What is the significance of the increased uptake of ^{99m}Tc sulphur colloid by the spleen.
2. What is the probable cause of this woman's painful soles?
3. Apart from painful soles, what are the other modes of presentation of this woman's problem?

Case 38

A 71-year-old man was admitted with a 2-month history of general physical deterioration and a 1-month history of confusion and increasing dependency. Several months earlier he had been diagnosed as having hypertension for which he was taking methyldopa and a thiazide diuretic. On examination he was confused and had signs of dehydration. In the chest he had clinical and radiological features of consolidation at both bases. An ECG revealed changes compatible with a recent anterior myocardial infarction.

Investigations

Glucose: 56.0 mmol/l
Potassium: 4.3 mmol/l
Sodium: 165 mmol/l
Urea: 38 mmol/l
Urinalysis: presence of glucose only

Questions

1. What are the diagnoses?
2. What are the probable precipitating factors responsible for the biochemical abnormalities?

3. How should the biochemical abnormalities be treated?
4. What is the prognosis in this patient.

Case 39

An 85-year-old man who lived with his wife on a top floor self-contained flat in his own house, was admitted with a 1-month history of increasing breathlessness, associated with ankle swelling, dysphagia and malaise. Although his dyspnoea was worse at night he had no attacks of PND. The dysphagia was worse when ingesting solids and was accompanied by a burning ache in the lower retrosternal region. In the past he had an attack of paroxysmal nodal tachycardia, and pulmonary TB many years earlier.

On examination he looked unwell, was cachectic and cyanosed. He had early finger clubbing, a regular pulse 96 beats/min and a blood pressure of 100/70 mmHg. Other significant findings were a raised JVP by 3 cm, displaced heart apex beat with fourth heart sound, signs of large left pleural effusion and an enlarged smooth liver 2 cm below the costal margin.

Investigations

Haemoglobin: 8.7 g/dl
MCV: 89 fl
WCC: 6.4×10^9/l
Serum iron: 5.5 μmol/l
TIBC: 73.5 μmol/l
ESR: 20 mm in first hour
Pleural fluid protein: 12 g/l
MSU: no growth
Blood culture: 3/6 produced growth of Diphtheroids

Albumin: 35 g/l
Alkaline phosphatase: normal
AST: 91 IU/l
Calcium: normal
Glucose: 6.6 mmol/l
Potassium: normal
Phosphate: normal
Random glucose: 6.7 mmol/l
Urea: 14.3 mmol/l
Vitamin B12: normal
Folic acid: normal

Echocardiogram: revealed large left atrium, thickened aortic valve with restricted opening but no vegetations
Barium meal: confirmed presence of large left atrium
Chest X-ray: showed pleural thickening at right apex and presence of left pleural effusion
ECG: showed sinus rhythm with lateral ischaemic changes.

Questions

1. What diagnoses would you make in this patient?
2. What is the cause of his dysphagia?
3. What treatment should he receive during admission?

Case 40

A 67-year-old woman, a known hypertensive for 7 years for which she was taking atenolol, presented with malaise and was found to have serum calcium of 2.84 mmol/l with an albumin of 40 g/l. Systems review revealed no other significant symptom. Clinical examination revealed a blood pressure of 160/105 mmHg and nothing else of note.

Questions

1. Which drugs would you enquire about in this patient?
2. What investigations would you carry out?
3. What are the 2 most likely diagnoses?
4. What is (are) the mechanism(s) of hypercalcaemia of malignancy?

Case 41

A 75-year-old woman was admitted to hospital following a fall due to a trip. In doing this she sustained a fracture to the right humerus. Clinical examination revealed signs of the fracture but nothing else.

Investigations

Haemoglobin: 8.6 g/dl
MCV: 110 fl
WCC: $13.8 \times 10^9/l$
Platelet count: $350 \times 10^9/l$
TIBC: normal
Serum iron: normal
Liver function tests: normal
Bone biochemistry: normal
Urea: normal
Electrolytes: normal
Vitamin B12: normal
Folic acid: normal

Bone marrow was hypercellular with all cell lines showing some morphological abnormalities. Not only were there some ring sideroblasts but myelocytes showed dysplasia. Iron stores were generally increased. Although serum B12 and serum folate were within normal limits the patient was given replacement therapy using these. After 3 months there was no change in the haemoglobin or the MCV.

Questions

1. What type of anaemia does this patient have?
2. How would you treat this patient?
3. List 5 causes of macrocytosis?

Case 42

A 74-year-old man who lived in his own house was admitted with a 1-week history of dysphagia and regurgitation. He had cerebral palsy at birth, anaemia secondary to oesophagitis in the past year and carcinoma of the rectum for which he had abdomino-perineal resection at approximately the same time.

On examination he was apyrexial but retching, with a pulse of 80 beats/min regular and blood pressure 170/80 mmHg. The other significant findings were signs of spastic quadroparesis (present since birth) and colostomy.

Investigations

Haemoglobin: normal	Alkaline phosphatase: 184 IU/l
WCC: normal	AST: 46 IU/l
	Calcium: normal
	Phosphate: normal
	Thyroxine: 132 nmol/l

X-ray of chest: revealed cardiomegaly with shadowing consistent with right lower lobe pneumonia, also an air fluid level behind the heart
Barium meal: confirmed the presence of a large hiatus hernia with the whole of the stomach lying rotated in the thorax.

Questions

1. What diagnoses would you make in this patient?
2. What was the cause of the painful dysphagia?
3. What are the complications of the condition that produces dysphagia and what treatment would you recommend to the patient?
4. What are the common motility disorders of the oesophagus that can cause dysphagia in the elderly?

Case 43

An 81-year-old woman was referred to the outpatient clinic with a 1-week history of spontaneous onset of mid-chest discomfort on swallowing food which was worse with liquids than with solids. She experienced a burning sensation on drinking hot liquids. This patient had lost 1 stone in weight over the previous year. There were no symptoms of aspiration or regurgitation and there was no history of blood loss from the gastrointestinal tract. At the time of review her treatment consisted of frusemide and potassium chloride tablets. Clinical examination revealed signs of mild CCF only.

Questions

1. What are the diagnostic possibilities?
2. Could drugs produce the symptoms this patient had?
3. What investigations should be carried out?

Case 44

An 84-year-old widower was admitted to hospital following progressive but general deterioration over many months. He had lived in the same ground floor flat since he was married and the condition of the flat at the time of admission was squalid. He himself was very reluctant to seek medical help partly through his personality and partly because of his embarrassment at his severe phimosis. He gave no other significant past medical history.

On examination he was dehydrated and looked uraemic. His respiratory rate was 44 beats/min, pulse 120 beats/min regular, blood pressure 80/60 mmHg. Heart sounds were normal and in the chest there was an occasional wheeze. The abdomen was soft and there were no obvious masses palpable although he was dull to percussion suprapubically up to the umbilicus. Rectal examination revealed presence of dark brown faeces. The prostate gland was not felt. He had tight phimosis with urinary incontinence.

Investigations

Haemoglobin: 11.4 g/dl
WCC: 16.6×10^9/l
Platelet count: normal

Acid phosphatase: normal
AST: marginally elevated
Amylase: 555 IU/l
Bicarbonate: 16.3 mmol/l
Bilirubin: marginally elevated

Urinary sodium: 12.0 mmol/l
Urinary urea: 68 mmol/l
Urinary osmolality: 627 mosm/kg
Plasma osmolality: 350 mosm/kg

Calcium: normal
Phosphate: normal
Random glucose: 8.2 mmol/l
Sodium: 165 mmol/l
Urea: 49.8 mmol/l
Thyroxine: normal
Vitamin B12: normal
Serum folate: normal
Red cell folate: normal

Ultrasound of abdomen: revealed large bladder and grossly hydronephrotic kidneys.

Questions

1. What are the probable diagnoses in this patient?
2. How would you treat this patient?
3. What discharge plans would you make for this man?

Case 45

A 67-year-old mentally subnormal woman, who lived alone was brought to hospital by neighbours who found her lying at the bottom of a flight of stairs. She had been epileptic since childhood and was taking phenobarbitone 30 mg tds.

On examination she was clinically anaemic, had a hoarse voice and bradycardia, but no peripheral oedema. Heart sounds were normal. She was fully conscious but totally disorientated in time and place, and there were no focal neurological signs.

Investigations

Haemoglobin: 8.6 g/dl
Plasma osmolality: 222 mmol

Potassium: 4 mmol/l
Sodium: 118 mmol/l

Total T4: 15 nmol/l
TSH: 62 mU/l
X-ray of skull: showed linear occipital fracture only.

Questions

1. Why was she hyponatraemic?
2. What would you do prior to instituting thyroxine replacement therapy?
3. Outline your treatment regimen?
4. What conditions are associated with slow-relaxing reflexes?

Case 46

An 87-year-old woman who lived with her daughter and son-in-law was admitted with acute onset of confusion. According to the daughter, during the 2 days prior to admission the patient had become agitated and at times was hallucinating. In addition she had become incontinent of urine. The symptoms were intermittent. At the time of admission she was disorientated in time and place but had a mental test score of 5 out of 10. Her pulse was 80 beats/min with multiple ectopic beats and a blood pressure of 160/90 mmHg. On auscultation she had a ejection systolic murmur and grade 2/6 early diastolic murmur. There were no focal neurological signs.

Investigations

Haemoglobin: 14.4 g/dl
WCC: 9×10^9/l
PCV: 45%
ESR: 10 mm in first hour

Urea: 10.5 mmol/l
Electrolytes: normal

Liver function tests: normal
Blood cultures: sterile
X-ray of chest: revealed cardiomegaly.

Questions

1. What is the probable cause of her confusion?
2. What treatment would you give this woman?
3. What are the common causes of urinary incontinence in the elderly?
4. What information would you give to the family about the patient's confusion?

Case 47

A 75-year-old retired engineer was admitted with a 12-hour history of severe colicky right upper quadrant pain. Since the onset of the pain, his bowels had been opened twice with the passage of normal stools. He denied vomiting and had no past history of abdominal pain. He lost his appetite 9 months previously when his wife died and had subsequently since lost over 1 stone in weight. On further questioning he gave a 2-week history of shortness of breath and ankle swelling.

On examination he was pyrexial, unwell but not clinically jaundiced. He had an irregular radial pulse of 140 beats/min with an apex rate of 200 beats/min, a blood pressure of 170/100 mmHg, a JVP raised by 10 cm and bilateral pitting oedema to the knees. His apex beat was displaced to the anterior axillary line and a gallop rhythm was heard. There were bilateral basal crackles in the chest. In the abdomen he was tender, with guarding in the right hypochondrium and the liver was palpable 3 cm below the costal margin. Rectal examination was unremarkable and bowel sounds were normal.

Investigations

Haemoglobin: normal
WCC: 15×10^9/l (with 82% neutrophils)

Alkaline phosphatase: 263 IU/l
Bilirubin: 23 μmol/l

Cardiac enzymes: normal

Calcium: normal
Gamma GT 80 IU/l
Phosphate: normal
Electrolytes: normal
Random blood glucose: normal

A diagnosis of acute cholecystitis and heart failure associated with atrial fibrillation was made and he was treated with antibiotics, digitalization and diuretics. Clinically the patient improved but, despite digitalization, he remained in rapid atrial fibrillation. At this stage results of his thyroid function tests came back and the values were as follows: T4 120 nmol/l (NR 55–155), free T4 74 pmol/l (NR 8–30) total T3 2.86 nmol/l (NR 0.8–2.5).

Questions

1. How would you interpret the results of the thyroid function tests?
2. Outline further management?
3. What are the possible causes for his initially abnormal liver function results?

Case 48

A 78-year-old woman, who lived with her husband in sheltered accommodation, was admitted following an acute onset of giddiness, facial numbness and diplopia. This episode resulted in a fall. Following this she developed pain in her left hip.

On examination she had a pulse of 80 beats/min regular, a blood pressure of 200/120 mmHg, with postural drop of 25 mmHg, left ventricular hypertrophy but normal heart sounds, diplopia on looking to right with mild ataxia of the right arm, gross truncal ataxia and dilated and tortous retinal veins on fundoscopy.

Investigations

Haemoglobin: 10.6 g/dl
WCC: 6.7 × 10^9/l
ESR: 136 mm in first hour with rouleaux formation

Albumin: 28 g/l
Alkaline phosphatase: 148 IU/l
Calcium: normal
Creatinine: 77 μmol/l
Gamma GT: 101 IU/l
Globulin: 72 g/l
Random glucose: 6.6 mmol/l
Potassium: 3.1 mmol/l
Phosphate: normal
Sodium: 125 mmol/l
Urea: 4.0 mmol/l

Protein electrophoresis: revealed the presence of a monoclonal band – IgA: 11.8 g/l, IgG: 0.54 g/l, IgM: 66.3 g/l
Chest X-ray: showed borderline cardiomegoly but lungs were clear
Skull X-rays: normal
Clotting studies: normal
Bone marrow lymphoid cells moderately increased but with no abnormal plasma cells
Whole blood viscosity: corrected to normal haematocrit at 230/s was 7.4 cps (NR 2.7–5.0) and at 23/s was 10.6 cps (NR 4.0–8.4).

During the next 2 weeks she developed bladder dysfunction with increased residual urine, extensive bruising and right superficial peroneal palsy. Regrettably her husband who had been taken into a home died 2 days after the move.

Questions

1. What is the diagnosis?
2. How would you treat this patient?
3. What is the prognosis in this woman?
4. In addition to medical treatment, what other plans would you make for this patient?

Case 49

An 81-year-old woman was admitted with a 1-week history of nausea, anorexia and lethargy. Three days earlier she had developed a productive cough for which her general practitioner had prescribed antibiotics. She had been discharged from hospital 2 weeks previously having been admitted with hypothermia and pneumonia. She was normally fully independent and lived with her daughter. On admission she was taking a mixture of amiloride and hydrochlorothiazide (Moduretic, once daily), and Gaviscon 10 ml bd. She drank stout occasionally and smoked 2 cigarettes per day.

On examination she was drowsy and cold but not shivering. Her rectal temperature was 33°C, pulse 56 beats/min regular and blood pressure 110/70 mmHg. There was pitting ankle oedema to the mid calf but no sacral pad. Heart sounds were normal with an ejection systolic murmur. Chest expansion was poor and she had impaired percussion note and coarse crackles at the left base. Abdominal examination was unremarkable apart from faecal impaction. She was extremely drowsy and confused. Reflexes in the upper limbs were sluggish and slow relaxing, but reflexes in the lower limbs were absent altogether. Both plantar responses were flexor.

Investigations

Haemoglobin: 10.9 g/dl
MCV: 99 fl
WCC: 3.9 × 10^9/l

Amylase: normal
Random blood glucose: 3.4 mmol/l
Potassium: 5.7 mmol/l
Sodium: 131 mmol/l

X-ray of chest: shadowing in left lower zone compatible with infection

A diagnosis of hypothermia and chest infection was made. She was gradually rewarmed, rehydrated and treated with antibiotics. Despite this, she remained hypothermic and 3 days later her electrolyte disturbances became more marked with sodium 119 mmol/l and potassium of 5.0 mmol/l.

Questions

1. Would rapid surface rewarming have been more appropriate in this case?
2. What are the causes of resistant hypothermia?
3. What are the possible causes of her initial hyponatraemia?
4. What further investigations are indicated?

Case 50

An 88-year-old woman who had had lumbar back pain for many years, was admitted because this had been worse during the week prior to admission. On the day of admission she had become confused. At this time she was taking frusemide 40 mg a day, Slow K ii tablets daily and indomethacin 50 mg tds.

On examination she appeared comfortable while lying on her back. Her pulse was 110 beats/min irregular and blood pressure 140/80 mmHg. Heart sounds I and II were normal. No abnormality was detected in the chest. In the abdomen she had minimal tenderness in the epigastrium but there were no palpable masses and the bowel sounds were normal. Rectal examination revealed soft motions of normal colour. Percussion of the lumbar spine revealed no pain.

Investigations

Radiology of chest and lumbar spine. Findings on X-ray of the chest led to her having an emergency surgical treatment.

Questions

1. What did the X-rays demonstrate to lead to emergency surgery?
2. What adjustments would you make to the therapy?

3. What treatment would you recommend for her thin, collapsed vertebrae?

Case 51

A 79-year-old man who lived with his wife and son was referred to the day hospital with deteriorating mobility. His complaint at the time was weakness in the legs, loss of appetite, pain in the lower dorsal spine and pain in the epigastric region which related to movement.

On examination the positive findings were pulse of 70 beats/min regular, blood pressure 120/80 mmHg, aortic sclerotic murmur, swelling of ankles and knees, enlarged prostatic gland, hyperaesthesia in D11/12 on left with a diffuse sensory level at approximately the same level on the left, muscle power reduced in both legs, absent left knee and right ankle jerks, reduced right knee and left ankle jerks but equivocal planters.

Investigations

Haemoglobin: 9.9 g/dl
WCC: 5.5 × 10^9/l (with 5% myelocytes and 1% nucleated red cells)

Acid phosphatase: 6.45 IU/l
Alkaline phosphatase: 140 IU/l
Sodium: 129 mmol/l
Electrolytes: normal

X-ray of dorsal spine: revealed areas of increased density in the lower dorsal vertebrae.

Questions

1. What are the probable diagnoses in this patient?
2. What treatment would you consider giving this patient?

3. What are the benign causes of leucoerythroblastic anaemia?

Case 52

An 85-year-old woman who lived with her sister and was supported by a home help was admitted with a few days history of increasing dyspnoea on exertion without orthopnoea. Prior to this, she had septicaemia a year earlier, and hypertension for many years for which she was taking a mixture of atenolol and chlorthalidone (Tenoretic) 1 tablet daily. She was also taking indomethacin for arthritic pain in the hips.

On examination she had a pulse of 70 beats/min regular, and blood pressure of 150/80 mmHg. The other significant features were those of left ventricular hypertrophy, aortic sclerotic murmur, bilateral crepitations at both bases and ankle oedema.

Investigations

Haemoblobin: 8.9 g/dl
MCV: 82 fl
WCC: $5.6 \times 10^9/l$

Urea: 13.5 mmol/l
Electrolytes: normal
Thyroxine: 81 µmol/l (normal)

Liver function tests: normal
ECG: confirmed presence of sinus rhythm with ST segment changes and T-wave inversion in leads I and aVl.
X-ray of chest: cardiomegaly, with shadowing at both lung bases.

The management consisted of stopping the Tenoretic and starting frusemide and amiloride. On this regime her symptoms improved but her urea climbed to 22 mmol/l and potassium rose to 8.1 mmol/l

Questions

1. What changes did the repeat ECG show?

2. What was the cause of this patient's hyperkalaemia?
3. What treatment did she receive?

Case 53

An 87-year-old widow living alone in a ground floor council flat was found on the floor by her daughter-in-law and admitted to hospital. At home she was supported by a home help twice weekly, a district nurse fortnightly and by her daughter-in-law who visited her every morning to help the patient with washing and dressing. Her past medical history was a cholecystectomy 50 years ago, a right hip fracture 6 years ago, arthritis of knees, hips, elbows and hands for many years and hypertension for several years for which she was taking bendrofluazide (1 tablet daily).

On examination she was mildly confused and although confabulating, she scored 5/10 on the Royal College of Physicians mental test score. In addition to this she had a large effusion of the left shoulder, a regular pulse of 92 beats/min, a blood pressure of 140/90 mmHg, tophi on many proximal and distal interphalangeal joints.

Investigations

Haemoglobin: 14.0 g/dl
WCC: 13.0×10^9/l
ESR: 10 mm in first hour

Random glucose: 7.0 mmol/l
Calcium: normal
Phosphate: normal
Thyroxine: 109 nmol/l
Urea: 8.4 mmol/l
Uric acid: 0.62 mmol/l
Electrolytes: normal

Liver function tests: normal

The chest X-ray was normal but the X-ray of left shoulder revealed fracture of left clavicle and surgical neck of left humerus with mild OA in the gleno-humeral joint. X-ray of the pelvis revealed an old trans-trochanteric fracture of right femur – although this had been treated with pin and plate, the femoral head had been resorbed over the last few years; X-rays of the hands revealed erosions with secondary osteoarthritic changes and soft tissue swellings.

Once her condition had improved and mobility achieved the patient expressed a desire to go home; however, her daughter-in-law refused to accept this and said that if she was discharged home she would not visit her again.

Questions

1. What are the possible causes of the shoulder effusion?
2. What is the condition that is affecting her hand joints?
3. How would you plan this woman's future care?

Case 54

A 75-year-old man, with a past history of hypertension and congestive cardiac failure and long-established chronic obstructive airways disease, was admitted with a frontal headache and a 4-day history of nausea and true vertigo. Additionally, he had noticed progressive weakness of his legs, dysarthria and ataxia. At the time of admission he was taking digoxin (0.125 mg daily), frusemide (40 mg daily). spironolactone (25 mg bd) and prochlorperazine (5 mg tds).

On examination the patient was a pleasant man, although somewhat dysarthric and had plethoric facies. His pulse was 80 beats/min in atrial fibrillation and his blood pressure 140/80 mmHg. Other signs were (i) a late systolic apical murmur without a click, (ii) the use of accessory muscles for respiration, (iii) diplopia with a mild right sixth nerve palsy, (iv) horizontal nystagmus, (v) mild right and possibly left facial weakness, (vi) dysphonia in addition to dysarthria, (vii) increased tone on the left side, (viii) bilateral mild pyramidal weakness, (ix) bilateral limb ataxia, (x) marginally brisk reflexes, (xi) extensor plantars on both sides and (xii) severe ataxia on walking.

Investigations

Haemoglobin: 19.6 g/dl
PCV: 62
WCC: 13×10^9/l (with predominance of polymorphs)
Platelet count: normal
Blood cultures: negative
Urea: 11.3 mmol/l
Random glucose: 15.5 mmol/l
Electrolytes: normal
Bone biochemistry: normal

MSU: clear
Liver function tests: normal
Cardiac enzymes: normal
Chest X-ray: showed cardiomegaly
ECG: atrial fibrillation with T wave insertion over S1, aVl and arterior leads III–VI in addition to multifocal ventricular ectopic beats.

Questions

1. What diagnoses would you make?
2. What are the possible factors that contributed to his neurological problem?
3. What would be the management of this patient?

Case 55

An 85-year-old retired man who lived alone was admitted with a 2-month history of increasing weakness of the left arm. Three weeks prior to admission he developed pain in the neck radiating to the back of the head and down the left arm and increasing difficulty in walking.

On examination the patient looked anaemic, had a regular pulse of 80 beats/min with occasional ectopic beats and blood pressure of 170/90 mmHg. Other signs were as follows: (i) bilateral ankle oedema, (ii) fasciculation of muscles of both upper limbs, (iii) global weakness of all muscles in the limbs, (iv) marked wasting of the deltoids especially on the left, (v) absent reflexes in the legs and arms (except for biceps jerk in the right arm, (vi) bilateral extensor plantar responses but without any sensory level and (viii) a large, hard prostate on PR examination.

Investigations

Haemoglobin: 9.2 g/dl
Serum iron: 11 μmol/l
TIBC: 82.5 μmol/l
ESR: 51 mm in first hour
1-h post-prandial blood glucose: 12 mmol/l
Protein electrophoretic strip: normal

Albumin: 38 g/l
Acid phosphatase: 34.4 IU/l
Alkaline phosphatase: 1320 IU/l
AST: 19 IU/l
Bilirubin: 3 μmol/l
Calcium: 2.19 mmol/l
Creatinine: 120 μmol/l
Phosphate: 0.50 mmol/l
Urea: normal
Electroytes: normal
24-h urine phosphate: 15.8 mmol/24-h

Skeletal survey: showed extensive Paget's disease with diffuse lytic destruction involving all the vertebrae (particularly cervical) leading to collapse.

Questions

1. What are the probable diagnoses in this patient?
2. What is the cause of hypophosphataemia in this patient, and what are the causes of profound hypophosphataemia in general?
3. What treatment did he receive?
4. What information would you give to the patient on discharge?

Case 56

A 79-year-old woman who lived alone in a ground floor flat was admitted following a fall which occurred 1 week earlier.

As a result, the patient had taken to bed and had become immobile. Three weeks previously she was discharged home from another hospital where she was admitted earlier with bronchopneumonia and heart failure. For this she was given a 10-day course of antibiotics. At the time of the second admission she was taking Frumil, digoxin and paracetamol.

On examination she looked well and had pulse of 104 beats/min in atrial fibrillation and a blood pressure of 100/60 mmHg. The remainder of the examination was essentially normal apart from a few crepitations at both bases in the chest, large ulcers on both ankles, a small superficial sacral sore and osteoarthritic changes in the knees.

Investigations

Normal apart from raised white cell count of 14.9×10^9/l and raised urea at 40.3 mmol/l. Chest X-ray showed resolving pneumonia. Two days after admission the patient developed diarrhoea. As a result sigmoidoscopy was carried out and this revealed patchy exudative membranes covering inflamed mucosa.

Questions

1. What is the likely cause of the patient's diarrhoea and how would you confirm the diagnosis?
2. What is the treatment and prognosis of this condition?
3. What would be your plan for future care of this woman?

Case 57

An 82-year-old widow who lived with her daughter was admitted with dyspnoea and bilateral ankle swelling of several months duration and also anorexia. She denied having any chest pain or palpitations.

On examination she was dyspnoeic at rest, had a regular

pulse of 72 beats/min and a blood pressure of 100/60 mmHg. The apex beat was displaced to mid axillary line and, on auscultation, she had a gallop rhythm and a short ejection systolic murmur heard maximally at left sternal edge. The JVP was raised to the angle of her jaws and she had abdominal signs of ascites and hepatomegaly. In the chest, fine crepitations were heard in both lung bases.

Investigations

Haemoglobin: 14.0 g/dl
ESR: 6 mm in first hour

Alkaline phosphatase: 159 IU/l
AST: 35 IU/l
Bilirubin: 29 mmol/l
Calcium: normal
HBD: 260 IU/l
Potassium: 3.4 mmol/l
Phosphate: normal
Sodium: 134 mmol/l
Thyroxine: normal
Urea: 8.5 mmol/l

Chest X-ray: enlarged heart with bilateral effusions
ECG: low voltage complexes with diffuse T wave changes in almost all leads.

Questions

1. What is the differential diagnosis?
2. What further investigation would you perform in this patient?
3. How would you treat this patient?

Case 58

A 75-year-old man who was living with his wife was referred for domiciliary assessment. The patient gave a 3-month history of anorexia, nausea and giddiness. Ten years earlier he had been diagnosed as having polymyalgia rheumatica, 6 years earlier he had had a CVA; he had also suffered from chronic obstructive airways disease and heart failure. As the patient's breathing had recently worsened, his general practitioner had increased the digoxin dosage from 0.25 mg daily to 0.25 mg bd 2 days prior to the request for the visit. At the time of the domiciliary visit he was taking frusemide 80 mg daily, digoxin 0.25 mg bd, aminophylline 100 mg bd, prednisolone 1–2 mg on alternate days, methyldopa 250 mg mane, ferrous sulphate 200 mg tds.

On examination the patient was a thin man with signs of dehydration. His pulse was an irregular 60 beats/min and his blood pressure was 130/80 mmHg. Heart sounds were normal except for a loud aortic systolic murmur. There was no ankle or sacral oedema and JVP was not raised. The only other findings on examination were a small superficial sore on the right buttock and generally brisk reflexes.

Investigations

Haemoglobin: 11.4 g/dl
WCC: 5.8 × 10^9/l
Platelet count: 101 × 10^9/l
ESR: 10 mm in first hour
Liver function tests: normal
MSU: sterile
Blood culture: no growth (on 3 cultures)

Albumin: 31 g/l
Calcium: normal
Potassium: 4.0 mmol/l
Phosphate: normal
Random glucose: 4.8 mmol/l
Urea: 11.1 mmol/l
Uric acid: 0.61 mmol/l

Chest X-ray: revealed cardiomegaly with prominent pulmonary arteries but no evidence of heart failure
Echocardiogram: revealed heavily calcified aortic valve with reduced opening, with some calcification of the mitral valve. The left ventricle was also dilated
ECG: showed atrial fibrillation and bigemini.

Questions

1. What was the main cause of this patient's medical condition?
2. How would you manage this patient?
3. Does he still require steroid treatment for the polymyalgia rheumatica?

Case 59

An 82-year-old man with a previous cerebrovascular accident, who was on a continuing care ward developed an eczematous rash involving the extensor surfaces. For this he was started on corticosteroid ointment, antihistamine for itching and flucloxacillin for the secondary infection on the advice of a consultant dermatologist. On this treatment his rash improved, but 3 weeks later he developed blisters on his hands and knees. Some of these burst easily and became infected.

Investigations

Haemoglobin: 10.9 g/dl
WCC: 11 300 (with 45% eosinophils)

Questions

1. What is the differential diagnosis in this patient?
2. How would you confirm the diagnosis?
3. What treatment will you give to this patient?
4. What are the causes of eosinophilia?

Case 60

An 80-year-old woman who was a non-smoker was admitted with a 1 week history of swelling of right calf. She denied having any chest pain or trauma to her leg.

On examination she looked well, but had a swollen right leg up to the thigh. She was tender on the left calf, and this leg felt warmer than the right.

Investigations

Urea: normal
Electrolytes: normal

Full blood count: normal
Random blood glucose: normal
Chest X-ray: normal
Abdominal ultrasound: normal
Liver function tests: normal
ECG: showed inferior ischaemic changes only

Clinical diagnosis of deep vein thrombosis were made and the patient was started on IV heparin for 10 days in addition to giving her elastic stockings. The dose of heparin was monitored with whole blood clotting studies. After 10 days, when the heparin had been stopped, she developed numbness of the left leg with weakness of quadriceps and depression of knee jerk. In addition, she had bruising on the left chest wall and a suggestion of a mass in the left groin.

Questions

1. What was the cause of her neurological symptoms and signs?
2. What treatment should she receive?

Part 2

Answers, Comments and References

Case 1

Answers

1. Temporal arteritis. Diagnosis can be confirmed by temporal artery biopsy.
2. Yes. Although value of the ESR is often more than 100 mm in the first hour, in patients with temporal arteritis it can be within normal limits.
3. Yes. Mild elevation of alkaline phosphatase and transaminases can be found in patients with temporal arteritis, and in these individuals malignancy may be erroneously suspected.
4. The 4 atypical presentations could result from any of the 7 causes listed below:
   (i) pyrexia of unknown origin,
   (ii) psychiatric (depression or dementia),
   (iii) involvement of other arteries leading to stroke, myocardial infarction, etc,
   (iv) Pseudoneoplastic syndrome (a patient with this often presents with vague ill-health, weight loss and anaemia),
   (v) renal involvement (nephritic urinary sediment with red cell casts; significant parenchymal involvement is rare),
   (vi) abnormal liver function and

(vii) normochromic normocytic anaemia.

5. The social services were asked by the general practitioner to provide care at home for the patient's 86-year-old husband. Services required were 'meals on wheels', 'home help' and the district nurse as well as help of a neighbour.

Discussion

In the elderly the ESR is a difficult test to interpret. Normal asymptomatic elderly people can have ESRs of 60 whereas sick elderly with severe infection or malignancy can have ESRs of less than 10 mm in the first hour.

Once the diagnosis of temporal arteritis is suspected, the patient should be given steroids to prevent blindness. It is important not to wait for the result of the temporal artery biopsy as histological changes can still be detected 7–10 days after starting the treatment.

Polymyalgia rheumatica is a manifestation of giant cell arteritis in 50% of cases. Its peak incidence is at 70–79 years of age accounting for about 1.3% of all cases presenting at a rheumatology clinic.

The clinical features of polymyalgia rheumatica are pain and stiffness in the pelvis and shoulder girdle, neck pain, muscle tenderness in the upper arms and thighs and synovitis and systemic symptoms.

Further reading

Coomes, E. N., Ellis, R. M. and Kay, A. G. 'A prospective study of 102 patients with the polymyalgia rheumatica syndrome', *Rheumatology and Rehabilitation* (1976), **15**, 270–276

Rai, G. S. 'Erythrocyte sedimentation rate and diseases in the elderly', *Journal of American Geriatric Society* (1979), **27**, 382–383

Sharland, D. E. 'Erythrocyte sedimentation rate: the normal range in the elderly', *Journal of American Geriatric Society* (1980), **28**, 346–348

Case 2

Answers

1. The probable diagnosis is Crohn's colitis, although carcinoma must be considered a possibility.
2. This can be confirmed by sigmoidoscopy and rectal biopsy.
3. Management of Crohn's colitis depends upon the severity of the condition. For a mild attack corticosteroid enemas with sulphasalazine are sufficient. For more severe attacks the use of oral prednisolone with or without azathioprine may be needed. The latter has been shown to reduce the dosage requirement for steroids in these patients. Controversy still persists as far as maintenance therapy or therapy during remission is concerned. Other agents that may be helpful in patients with concomitant large bowel disease are metronidazole and sulphasalazine. Metronidazole is useful especially if there is associated sepsis. Surgery is indicated if medical treatment fails or if complications such as fistulae develop.

   Colostomy has also been a useful adjunct to rest the bowel in patients who do not respond as quickly as expected to medical treatment.

   In addition to medical treatment, this patient may require rehabilitation to improve her mobility which would have ultimately deteriorated after protracted illness.

Discussion

Although Crohn's disease is most commonly seen in younger patients, it can occur in the elderly. Diagnosis should be considered in any elderly patient presenting with unexplained systemic symptoms, gastrointestinal symptoms (particularly diarrhoea) or anal symptoms.

Some workers have found elderly patients to have ileal disease often requiring multiple operations with high mortality; however, others have found that this disease more frequently presents with granulomatous colitis which rarely requires surgical intervention. The prognosis for elderly patients with distal colonic disease is good.

Further Reading

Rhodes, J. and Rose, J., 'Crohn's disease in the elderly', *British Medical Journal* (1985), **291,** 1149–1150

Tchirkow, G., 'The differential diagnosis of Crohn's disease in the geriatric patient', *Geriatric Medicine Today* (1985), **4,** 74–80

Case 3

Answers

1 (i) Rheumatoid arthritis,
   (ii) Anaemia,
   (iii) Felty's syndrome,
   (iv) Hiatus hernia,
   (v) Cellulitis of the legs.

2. The cause of the abnormal liver scan is Felty's syndrome associated with rheumatoid arthritis. The patient probably has nodular regenerative hyperplasia.
3. Management includes:
   (i) transfusion to correct anaemia,
   (ii) treatment of hypersplenism with drugs (e.g. gold, penicillamine, chloroquine) or by splenectomy. Both treatment modalities improve neutropenia and decrease the incidence of infection; however, splenectomy is not to be recommended lightly as there is a high postoperative mortality.
   (iii) rehabilitation. This includes treatment of her fear to stand or walk following a fall (ptophobia), and may require behavioural desensitization in combination with physical therapy.
   (iv) a visit prior to discharge by an occupational therapist.

Discussion

Not all cases of rheumatoid arthritis in the elderly are chronic. Approximately one third present with acute arthritis for the first time.

Felty's syndrome (i.e. splenomegaly, leucopenia and rheumatoid arthritis) was described by Felty in 1924. Although anaemia and thrombocytopenia, or both, can be present, they are not necessary for diagnosis. In addition to the above features, patients tend to have loss of weight, positive serology for arthritis, increased pigmentation and leg ulcers. Recently, liver disease in association with Felty's syndrome has been described. The common abnormality found on histological examination of the liver is nodular regenerative hyperplasia.

Anaemia associated with rheumatoid arthritis can be normochromic normocytic or hypochromic microcytic. The latter commonly results from gastrointestinal bleeding and ulceration from a non-steroidal anti-inflammatory drug.

Further Reading

Thorne, C., Urowitz, M. B., Wanless, I., Roberts, E. and Blendis, L. M., 'Liver disease in Felty's syndrome', *The American Journal of Medicine* (1982), **73**, 35–40

Case 4

Answers

1. The diagnosis is pseudogout and this can be confirmed by examination of synovial fluid where calcium pyrophosphate dihydrate crystals are usually found, as well as in polymorphonuclear leucocytes. These crystals are positively birefringent when viewed in a polaroid light microscope, whereas the urate crystals found in gout are negatively birefringent.
2. Conditions which can be associated with pseudogout are:
   (i) gout,
   (ii) hyperparathyroidism,
   (iii) haemochromatosis,
   (iv) hypothyroidism,
   (v) diabetes mellitus,

(vi) amyloid,
(vii) trauma, and
(viii) steroid therapy.

3. The treatment of an acute attack is by the use of anti-inflammatory agents like indomethacin or azapropazone or, possibly, colchicine in some patients. Acute attacks may also be controlled by aspiration of the effusion. There is no maintenance therapy required and each attack is treated with a non-steroidal anti-inflammatory drug. Allopurinol is ineffective.
4. Raised bilirubin levels may have resulted from *in vitro* haemolysis or illness. The reasons for a raised bilirubin value during a serious illness in the elderly are poorly understood.

Discussion

Pseudogout presents acutely and is very painful. There is an intense inflammatory reaction with pus cells (polymorphs) in large numbers; thus infective arthritis may be diagnosed in error. Microscopic examination for organisms and culture of fluid should therefore be carried out to exclude such diagnoses in patients with swollen knees.

Further Reading

McCarty, D., 'Crystals, joints and consternation', *Annuals of the Rheumatic Diseases* (1983), **42,** 243–253

Dieppe, P. A., *'Examination of synovial fluid',* Report on Rheumatic diseases, Arthritis and Rheumatism Council (1983), No 83

Case 5

Answers

1. Important details that need to be ascertained include:
   (i) the relationship of symptoms to palpitations, to posture and to neck turning,

(ii) the presence of brainstem symptoms,
(iii) the relationship of symptoms to coughing or micturition
(iv) drug history and
(v) the presence of abnormal sweating, nocturnal diarrhoea or retention of urine which might indicate autonomic neuropathy.

2. The R–R interval response to the valsalva manoeuvre and changes in posture (supine to standing or standing to supine) as well as the 30/15 ratio (see below*). In this case there was no change in the R–R interval with normal respiration or valsalva manoeuvre, and the 30/15 ratio was 1. These changes were highly suggestive of autonomic neuropathy.
3. Treatment is often difficult and unsatisfactory; however, the following regimen may prove helpful:
   (i) remove any underlying precipitating cause i.e. offending drugs, correct dehydration and anaemia,
   (ii) instruct patient to change his posture slowly,
   (iii) keep head and trunk elevated at night thus promoting renin release and vascular expansion,
   (iv) give the patient supportive garments (e.g. stockings),
   (v) use drug therapy in the form of fludrocortisone to expand the intravascular volume. The starting dose should be 0.1 mg daily, and this should be increased slowly. Other agents that have been tried with some success include phenylephrine, prostaglandin synthesase inhibitors, β-blockers (of which pindolol is the most promising, especially in those with supine hypertension). Combinations of these drugs are also sometimes effective.

*If the R–R interval at beat 30 is divided by that at beat 15 a ratio of 1 or less is found in those patients with autonomic neuropathy.

Discussion

Syncope is a common problem in the elderly because of age-related physiological and disease-related changes. Questioning about past medical history should include details of drug history and the nature of onset. Physical examination should be devoted to the exclusion of postural hypotension, hypertrophic obstructive cardiomyopathy, aortic stenosis and carotid stenosis.

A 24-hour ECG record is commonly used as a diagnostic test; however, this is insensitive and there is poor correlation between findings and symptoms. Sick sinus syndrome is a major cause of syncope and, while it is associated with potential risk of morbidity, the 5-year survival is similar to normal age and sex-matched population. A pacemaker is indicated when concomitant sick sinus syndrome is present.

A condition often overlooked in the elderly is carotid sinus hypersensitivity. This is potentially treatable by insertion of a pacemaker or by the use of anti-cholinergic drugs. There are currently 2 types of carotid sinus hypersensitivity, namely cardioinhibitory and vasodepressor pacemakers.

Carotid sinus hypersensitivity can be diagnosed by performing carotid sinus massage, after confirming that there is no carotid bruit by auscultation. An abnormal result is indicated by cardiac asystole lasting more than 3 seconds, and a decrease in systolic blood pressure of 50 mmHg in association with symptoms, or both. Drugs (e.g. digitalis, propranolol and methyldopa) may produce an abnormal result.

Normal individuals have a tachycardia maximum around the fifteenth beat after standing up and relative bradycardia at around the thirtieth beat.

Further Reading

Schatz, J., 'Orthostatic hypotension: 11. Clinical, diagnosis, testing and treatment', *Archives of Internal Medicine* (1984), **144,** 1037–1041

Lipsitz, L. A., 'Syncope in the elderly', *Annals of Internal Medicine* (1983), **99,** 92–105

Sugrue, D. D., Wood, D. L. and McGoon, M. D., 'Cardiovascular clinics: catotid sinus hypersensitivity and syncope', *Mayo Clinic Proceedings* (1984), **59,** 637–640

Ewing, D. J., Campbell, I. W., Murray, A., Neilson, J. M. M. and Clarke, B. F., 'Immediate heart-rate response to standing: simple test for autonomic neuropathy in diabetes', *British Medical Journal* (1983), **1,** 145–147

Case 6

Answers

1. Subdural haematoma.
2. Head injury and alcohol.
3. No. Although confusion and particularly fluctuating drowsiness may occur, the most common symptom exhibited by patients is headache. The other modes of presentation include mild hemiparesis, aphasia, epilepsy, dementia or symptoms and signs of a mass lesion.

Discussion

Although a CT scan is the investigation of choice, the diagnosis may be made using an isotope brain scan. Diagnosis is indicated by the 'crescent' sign. In the case of a deteriorating clinical picture exploratory burrholes may be necessary.

Further Reading

Luxon, L. M. and Harison, M. J. G., 'Chronic subdural haematoma', *Quarterly Journal of Medicine* (1979), **189,** 43–53

Case 7

Answers

1. (i) Chronic active hepatitis associated with ulcerative colitis,
   (ii) Hepatitis secondary to diclofenac,
   (iii) Diabetes mellitus,
   Only (i) and (ii) need to be confirmed and this may be possible by carrying out a liver biopsy.
2. (i) Discontinue diclofenac therapy since this is known to affect liver function,

(ii) Administer a trial of steroids for chronic active hepatitis if her liver function tests remain abnormal despite the discontinuation of diclofenac.

Discussion

Although the changes revealed on biopsy were compatible with chronic active hepatitis, the liver function test results began to improve after the diclofenac therapy was stopped. Even the smooth muscle antibodies disappeared in 2 months. However, despite this the repeat liver biopsy showed no changes from the previous histology.

Changes of chronic active hepatitis can be produced by several drugs including methyldopa, isoniazid, nitrofurantoin, oxyphenistan and ketoconazole. These side-effects are more frequently seen in elderly patients.

Although chronic active hepatitis is predominantly a disease of younger people (particularly female) there is another peak incidence around the menopause. When associated with ulcerative colitis, chronic active hepatitis may not be apparent at presentation and may follow later. Treatment with steroids should only be given to those with symptoms, because of the many risks of steroid therapy including reactivation of tuberculosis. The course of the disease and prognosis are variable.

Further Reading

Woolf, I. Z., Boyes, B. E., Leeming, J. T. and Dymock, I. W., 'Active chronic hepatitis in the elderly', *Age and Ageing* (1974), **3**, 226–228

Joske, P. A., 'Active chronic hepatitis' *Modern Trends in Gastroenterology* (1975), **5**, 418–433. Butterworth, London

Case 8

Answers

1. A history of pruritus with dark urine and pale stools is

suggestive of obstructive jaundice. The differential diagnosis rests between a carcinoma arising from the head of the pancreas, bile duct or gallbladder and that of gallstones. In this patient the painless jaundice was suggestive of the former, despite the fact that the gallbladder was not palpable. However, it was possible that the jaundice may have been due to primary biliary cirrhosis or to prochlorperazine.

2. (i) Ultrasound examination of liver, gallbladder and biliary tract.
   (ii) If ducts are dilated on ultrasound consider ERCP or percutaneous cholangiography with or without laparotomy.
   (iii) If ducts are normal consider liver biopsy.

In this patient, ultrasound examination showed a dilated biliary tree and the presence of gallstones in an undilated gallbladder. Consequently, the patient had a laparotomy during which she was found to have a large tumour arising from the gallbladder which was invading the duct and the liver. Since a draining operation could not be carried out to relieve the obstruction, the patient was therefore referred for ERCP. During this an endoprosthesis was inserted using a torque stable guide. Her jaundice subsequently settled and she was discharged home with full community services and regular visits from a nurse.

Discussion

Carcinoma of the gallbladder is a disease of elderly females with an incidence of 0.2–5%. There is a close association of this tumour with the presence of gallstones. Stones with inflammation and infection are thought to contribute to the development of the tumour, which usually presents insidiously with weight loss, persistent right upper quadrant pain and jaundice. On examination, there is usually a hard mass in the right hypochondrium; however, this was not the case in our patient. Jaundice usually only appears when the disease is very advanced. ERCP shows irregular filling defects within the gallbladder.

Further Reading

Kelly, K. R. and Chamberlain, T. R., 'Carcinoma of the gallbladder', *The American Journal of Surgery* (1928), **143**, 737–741

Vallon, A. G., Croker, J. R., 'Obstructive jaundice in the elderly', *Age and Ageing* (1985), **14**, 143–148

Case 9

Answers

1. The diagnostic possibilities are:
   (i) primary slowly-resolving pneumonia,
   (ii) secondary pneumonia due to atypical organism,
   (iii) carcinoma with pneumonic consolidation and
   (iv) tuberculosis.
2. (i) Full screen for tuberculosis.
   (ii) Sputum sample for cytological examination.
   (iii) Serum examination for detection of antibodies to atypical organisms (e.g. *Mycoplasma, Legionella,* and *Psittaci).*
   (iv) Tomograms of his left upper lobe with or without CT scan of chest. In this case a CT scan of the chest revealed that the upper left chest was occupied by a soft tissue mass with mediastinal lymphadenopathy. Aspiration of a lymph node revealed an undifferentiated large cell carcinoma.
3. One could either continue the previous antibiotic for a longer period or introduce an agent like erythromycin to cover atypical infection. If this has no effect a trial of anti-tuberculosis therapy should be considered, provided that other causes, particularly malignancy, have been excluded by previous investigations.
4. Confusion accompanying any physical illness in the elderly is common. The most likely causes in this case are:
   (i) infection,
   (ii) secondary deposit in the brain,
   (iii) non-metastatic manifestation of carcinoma and
   (iv) metabolic disturbances. In this case a secondary deposit was an offending agent.

Discussion

Large cell carcinoma of lung is difficult to treat since the majority of cases are in elderly patients and most have metastases at diagnosis. Treatment of symptoms is all that can be offered. Combination chemotherapy in those patients with small cell carcinoma of lungs prolongs survival both in those with limited and widespread disease. This mode of therapy is, however, very toxic with an added risk of producing neurological syndromes. The risks have to be balanced against benefits.

Further Reading

Spiro, S. G., 'Editorial. Chemotherapy for small cell lung cancer', *British Medical Journal* (1985), **290**, 413–414

Case 10

Answers

1. An urticarial rash can be caused by multiple factors and these include:
   (i) allergy to drugs,
   (ii) insect bites,
   (iii) ingestion of certain foods particularly eggs, shellfish, nuts, strawberries,
   (iv) bacterial infection, (e.g. with *Streptococcus*),
   (v) viral infection,
   (vi) hereditary angioneurotic oedema,
   (vii) physical agents (e.g. 'cold'),
   (viii) emotional stress and
   (ix) neoplasms with or without cryoglobulinaemia.
   The diagnosis in this patient was angioneurotic oedema.
2. The abdominal symptoms of nausea, vomiting, abdominal pain and distension are suggestive of an obstruction; this may occur in patients with hereditary angioneurotic oedema because of oedema of the bowel wall. The X-rays

in this patient, however, suggested the presence of sigmoid volvulus. This was confirmed at sigmoidoscopy.

3. (i) The level of C_1 esterase inhibitor, which is a component of complement, is low in approximately 60% of cases of hereditary angio-oedema. The level was normal in this case.
   (ii) Cryoglobulins may be present, particularly in those with urticaria resulting from physical agents (e.g. 'cold') and in those with underlying lymphoproliferative states.
4. The usual symptomatic treatment of urticaria is not very successful in angioneurotic oedema. Skin involvement needs no treatment but acute attacks involving the airway may be life-threatening and should be treated with subcutaneous adrenaline and steroids. Aminocaproic acid may be of benefit in the long-term management to inhibit C_1 activation. Fresh frozen plasma and androgens have also been shown to be of benefit in these patients.

Case 11

Answers

1. (i) Paget's disease.
   (ii) Degenerative joint disease with lumbar spondylolisthesis.
   (iii) Possible osteomalacia secondary to gastrectomy suggested by low calcium.
2. (i) Fractures.
   (ii) Neurological complications – spinal cord and nerve root or cranial nerve compression, internal hydrocephalus, cerebellar involvement, etc.
   (iii) High output congestive cardiac failure.
   (iv) Neoplastic change to sarcoma.
   (v) Hypercalcaemia especially on immobilization.
3. (i) Symptomatic treatment: analgesia for pain.
   (ii) Specific treatment: calcitonin which inhibits bone

resorption. The dose should be 50–100 units daily for 1 month, and then reduced to 3 times per week. Treatment should be continued for at least 12 months.

The other drugs that could be tried in this condition are diphosphonates and mithramycin.

Discussion

Paget's disease is a common bone disorder affecting approximately 2–4% of those over the age of 60 years. The majority of patients with the disease are asymptomatic. Those with extensive disease may present with apathy and lethargy as well as bone pain and complications. The bones which are commonly involved are the skull, pelvis, sacrum, scapulae, spine and long bones.

Further Reading

Hamdy, R. C., *'Paget's Disease of Bone: Assessment and Management'*, Fletcher and Son, Norwich (1981)

Case 12

Answers

1. Asthma.
2. (i) Drowsiness and confusion due to CO_2 retention and hypoxia,
   (ii) pulsus paradoxicus,
   (iii) tachypnoea,
   (iv) tachycardia and
   (v) use of accessory muscles
3. Compliance may be a problem particularly with the use of bronchodilators (inhalers) because of difficulty of use. This can be improved by using nebuhalers, spacers or rotahalers, or aids to improve the delivery of an inhalation (e.g. Haleraid).

Discussion

The prevalence of asthma in the elderly is approximately 6.5%. The diagnosis is often missed because of:
(i) the coexistence of symptoms of chronic bronchitis,
(ii) the patient's lack of history of atopy or exercise-induced bronchospasm,
(iii) it is not appreciated that it can occur for the first time in the elderly, and
(iv) difficulty in obtaining and interpreting lung function tests in the elderly.

As in younger or middle aged patients, the elderly asthmatics can have severe acute exacerbation. Treatment should also be the same (i.e. inhaled bronchodilators with intravenous and oral corticosteroids). Of the many inhaled bronchodilators, ipratropium bromide has been suggested to be more effective in older patients. Some studies have shown that the absorption and elimination of theophilline is unaffected by age, but if the patient has taken theophilline prior to admission then blood concentrations should be performed, particularly to monitor the dosage. Eosinophilia may be present in blood and sputum, and in one series 50% of patients had eosinophilia.

Further Reading

Petheram, I. S., Jones, D. A. and Collins, J. V., 'Assessment and management of acute asthma in the elderly: a comparison with younger asthmatics', *Postgraduate Medical Journal* (1982), **58**, 149–151

Case 13

Answers

1. Acute confusional state in a patient with dementia. The cause for this in our patient was urinary tract infection.
2. The treatable causes one should consider and exclude can be any of the following:

  (i) subdural haematoma,
  (ii) depression (pseudodementia),
  (iii) normal pressure hydrocephalus,
  (iv) hypothyroidism,
  (v) vitamin B12 deficiency and
  (vi) folic acid deficiency.
3. Reduced choline acetyl transferase activity.

Discussion

This woman's long history of confusion and the absence of focal neurological signs is in keeping with a diagnosis of 'true' dementia. However, whenever there is a history of falls one must bear in mind the possibility of a subdural haemorrhage.

Depression often presents in the elderly as 'pseudodementia' with apathy, psychomotor retardation, impaired concentration, delusions and confusion. It usually has a shorter history than dementia and the patient usually complains of memory impairment, in contrast to dementia there is usually little insight into the degree of cognitive defect – except in early stages.

The diagnosis is made more difficult by the fact that up to 30% of demented patients are also depressed. If there is any doubt about the diagnosis, antidepressive treatment should be started.

Further Reading

Small, G. W. and Jarvik, L. F., 'The dementia syndrome', *Lancet* (1982), **II**, 1443–1446
Carnay, M, 'Pseudodementia', *British Journal of Hospital Medicine* (1983), **29**, 312–318

Case 14

Answers

1. Chronic renal failure: indicated by the presence of

anaemia, elevated phosphate and depressed serum calcium. He also has congestive cardiac failure.

2. Evidence of vasculitis and connective tissue disorders (e.g. lupus and polyarteritis nodosa) and band keratopathy which might indicate hyperparathyroidism.
3. The causes of chronic renal failure are similar to those in younger adults and include:
   (i) obstructive uropathy,
   (ii) interstitial nephritis,
   (iii) multiple myeloma,
   (iv) nephrotic syndrome,
   (v) connective tissue disease,
   (vi) metabolic conditions (e.g. diabetes mellitus, amyloidosis, hypercalcaemia),
   (vii) polycystic renal disease,
   (viii) nephrocalcinosis,
   (ix) glomerulonephritis and
   (x) analgesic nephropathy.

   In this case it was polycystic renal disease diagnosed on ultrasound.
4. The cause of his pericardial rub is uraemia.
5. The most important management step in this type of presentation is to decide whether one is dealing with a surgical or medical condition resulting in chronic renal failure. This can easily be ascertained by abdominal ultrasound. If there is evidence of obstruction, the treatment is surgical.

   If surgery is inappropriate the course of action is firstly to seek and treat any underlying cause especially infection, hypertension and dehydration as they are likely to produce deterioration in renal function leading to acute on chronic failure.

   Secondly dialysis should be performed, in view of the pericarditis followed by protein restriction. Vitamin D and a phosphate resin binder should then be administered.

   Although the elderly tolerate haemodialysis reasonably well continuous ambulatory peritoneal dialysis (CAPD) is perhaps an ideal modality of treatment for them.

Discussion

There are 2 types of polycystic renal disease:

(i) an infantile type with a recessive inheritance, and

(ii) adult type with a dominant inheritance.

The adult type can present at any age – even in the very elderly, in whom it may be found unsuspectedly at post mortem. It is therefore clear that, in some patients, the condition may follow a normal life expectancy.

The presenting features of this disease include hypertension, loin pain, chronic renal failure, haematuria, urinary tract infection and headache. In addition, patients may present with the discovery of an enlarged liver or pain due to bleeding into a cyst. These can occur in other organs such as the pancreas and lung. There is an increased prevalence of berry aneurysms and, in one study, a systolic murmur of unknown cause was noted.

There is no specific treatment for polycystic renal disease and management is directed towards the complications. One of the main tenets of management is genetic counselling; however, there is no reliable way of diagnosing the condition before the victim enters the reproductive period of life. Currently, ultrasound is the best method of investigation but its sensitivity depends on the age of patient. Recent genetic developments offer hope of earlier diagnosis.

Further Reading

Sahney, S., Sandler, M. A., Weiss, L., Levin, N. W., Hricak, H. and Madrazo, B. L., 'Adult polycystic kidney disease: presymptomatic diagnosis for genetic counselling', *Clinical Nephrology* (1983), **20,** 89–93

Reeders, S. T., Breuning, M. H., Corney, G., Jeremiah, S. J., Meera Khan, P., Davies, K. C., Hopkinson, D. A., Pearson, P. L. and Weatherall, D. J., 'Two genetic markers closely linked to adult polycystic kidney disease on chromosome 16', *British Medical Journal* (1986), **292,** 851–853

Case 15

Answers

1. Osteomalacia associated with phenobarbitone. Other factors that probably also contributed to the development of

osteomalacia in this woman include diet, lack of sunlight and living alone.
2. By bone biopsy.
3. On bone scan one may see generalized increased uptake with or without focal uptake by anterior ends of ribs, increased uptake at the costochondral junctions, 'tie sternum sign' and 'faint kidney sign' reflecting reduced excretion of tracer by kidneys due to increased skeletal uptake.
4. (i) Wean off barbiturates.
   (ii) Give vitamin D supplements.
   (iii) As the patient had been living alone in a large house a home visit from an occupational therapist would be required.

Discussion

Osteomalacia is common in the elderly and is reported to be present in approximately 4% of those admitted to a geriatric unit. Subclinical osteomalacia, however, is present in higher numbers.

The symptoms of osteomalacia include vague and generalized aches and pains, low backache, muscle weakness, waddling gait, bone pain and tenderness.

The aetiology is often multifactorial; however, factors that may play significant role are:
(i) inadequate intake of vitamin D,
(ii) lack of sunlight,
(iii) malabsorption,
(iv) gastrectomy,
(v) impaired hydroxylation of cholecalciferol,
(vi) increased catabolism of vitamin D and renal impairment leading to impaired conversion of 1, 25-dihydroxycholecalciferol to 1, 25-dihydroxycholecalciferol. In this patient it is probable that factors like living alone, poor diet and lack of sunlight all contributed to the development of osteomalacia.

Treatment comprises vitamin D adminstration and correction of the factors important in the aetiology of the condition. Vitamin D can be given orally in dose of 1000–1500 IU daily for 1 to 3 months or vitamin D with calcium tablets (1 bd). Those who are unlikely to comply with this treatment can be given parenteral therapy.

Further Reading

Fogelman, I., McKslop, J. H., Bessent, R. G., Boyle, I. T., 'Bone scanning in osteomalacia', *Journal of Nuclear Medicine* (1978), **19**, 245–248

Dent, C. E., Richens, A., Rowe, D. J. F. and Stamp, T. C. B., 'Osteomalacia with long term anticonvulsant therapy in epilepsy', *British Medical Journal* (1970), **4**, 69–72

Case 16

Answers

1. Bacterial meningitis from presumed infection of the middle ear.
2. Penicillin and gentamicin with intravenous fluids until the organism had been isolated from CSF and blood. In this patient *Streptococcus pneumoniae* was isolated from the blood, therefore the gentamicin was stopped after 36 hours.

Discussion

In the elderly with meningitis, neck stiffness when present may be confused with cervical spondylosis. A raised temperature, and increased WCC, as found in other infections, can be absent, and the mental changes may appear to be secondary to cerebrovascular disease. Although *Streptococcus pneumoniae* and *Neisseria meningitidis* are the predominant causative organisms, Gram negative bacilli and unusual pathogens such as *Listeria* should be considered. Therefore before administering empirical therapy for presumptive diagnosis of bacterial meningitis in the elderly, one must take into consideration these facts. The morbidity and mortality associated with this condition is high.

Further Reading

Norman, D. C. and Yoshikawa, T. T., 'Recognizing bacterial

meningitis in the elderly', *Geriatric Medicine Today* (1984), **3**, 85–88

Gorse, G., Thrupp, L. D. and Nudelman, K. L., 'Bacterial meningitis in the elderly', *Archives of Internal Medicine* (1984), **144**, 1603–1607

Case 17

Answers

1. High protein content suggests that the effusion is an exudate which can be produced by either pneumonia, malignancy, pulmonary infarction, collagen vascular disease, subphrenic abscess, Meigs syndrome or tuberculosis. The presence of lymphocytes in the absence of other features suggests that the cause is probably tuberculosis, this was confirmed by a growth of AFBs on culture of fluid.
2. The negative sputum examination for AFBs and the negative Mantoux test does not exclude tuberculosis. The Mantoux test is of little value in the elderly.
3. It is unlikely that treatment of the effusion will improve her mental impairment, particularly as history of increasing confusion for many years suggests presence of dementia in this patient.

Discussion

Tuberculosis is one of the infections whose incidence is increasing in the elderly while it is falling in the younger population. The clinical presentation of disease is often atypical in that classical features such as fever, sweats or cough are absent. Often these patients present with 'failure to thrive' at home, and often their chest X-rays are normal ('cryptic' tuberculosis). A high index of suspicion is thus required in these cases.

Isolation of the organism from sputum is often difficult and positive culture for AFBs may only be obtained from pleural biopsy, bone marrow or liver biopsy specimens in some patients.

Further Reading

Fullertan, J. M. and Dyer, L., 'Unsuspected tuberculosis in the aged', *Tubercle* (1965), **46**, 193–198
Rudd, A., 'Tuberculosis in a geriatric unit', *Journal of American Geriatric Society* (1985), **33**, 566–567

Case 18

Answers

1. (i) Diuretic therapy,
   (ii) malabsorption secondary to bacterial overgrowth as indicated by the abnormal breath test.
2. Only an ST wave depression was noted, the other changes of tall U waves and prolongation of the PR interval were not obvious on an ECG when the patient's heart rate was 160 beats/min.
3. She was given tetracycline for sterilization of her bowel.

Discussion

When elderly patients who have been taking diuretics for a long time develop hypokalaemia, other causes should be looked for, particularly loss of potassium through the gut. It is also possible that more than one cause is present in these patients.

In addition to cardiac conduction defects (especially in those with myocardial ischaemia or in those taking digoxin) hypokalaemia can lead to apathy, non-specific weakness due to myopathy, confusion, paralytic ileus and features of renal tubular damage.

In addition to hypokalaemia the use of diuretics in the elderly (particularly thiazides) can lead to urinary incontinence, acute retention, precipitation of diabetes mellitus and gout.

Further Reading

'Editorial: Diuretics in the elderly', *British Medical Journal* (1981), **1**, 1092–1093

Case 19

Answers

1. The most likely cause for her renal failure is massive procidentia causing obstructive uropathy and chronic pyelonephritis, or both.
2. With correction of the prolapse, renal function could return to normal.
3. Urinary tract infection.
4. Uraemia.

Discussion

Renal tract abnormalities associated with procidentia are common. Obstructive uropathy is present in 40% of those with third degree prolapse, this risk being related to the severity of the prolapse. Procidentia is also associated with a greatly increased incidence of recurrent urinary tract infection.

If correction of the prolapse is undertaken early enough (i.e. before the development of obstructive atrophy or chronic pyelonephritis) renal tract anatomy and renal function may return completely to normal.

Further Reading

Wright, G., Murphy, P. and Rai, G. S., 'Uterine prolapse: 12 cases show the need for action', *Geriatric Medicine* (1986), **16**, 49–52

Case 20

Answers

1. (i) Chronic lymphatic leukaemia.
   (ii) Herpes zoster involving T1 and T2.
   (iii) Congestive cardiac failure.
2. The 3 probable factors responsible for the pleural effusion are congestive cardiac failure, infection and leukaemic infiltration. In this patient, leukaemic infiltration was found of cytology of the pleural fluid.
3. The future complications likely to be experienced by this patient are:
   (i) post-herpetic neuralgia,
   (ii) side-effects of her cytotoxic therapy,
   (iii) blast crisis,
   (iv) haemolytic anaemia and
   (v) recurrent infections.

Discussion

The incidence of herpes zoster increases markedly with age. The precipitating factors include:
(i) trauma,
(ii) radiotherapy to the spinal cord,
(iii) malignancy,
(iv) chronic lymphatic leukaemia,
(v) lymphoma and
(vi) myeloma.
However, it is important to remember that herpes zoster can occur in patients without any of the above factors.

Treatment consists of 40% idoxuridine dissolved in DMSO, in the very early stages of the condition to relieve pain and to reduce post-hepatic neuralgia. Amantadine hydrochloride or acyclovir has also been found to be useful but the acyclovir has not been found to prevent post-hepatic neuralgia – a complication that particularly affects the elderly.

Further Reading

Hope-Simpson, R. E., 'The nature of herpes zoster: a long

term study and a new hypothesis', *Proceedings of the Royal Society of Medicine* (1965), **58**, 9–20

Case 21

Answers

1. The conditions to consider in differential diagnosis are gout, pseudogout, rheumatoid arthritis (RA), haemarthrosis, traumatic effusion and infection.
2. (i) to aspirate the effusion to obtain fluid for microscopy, Gram stain, for examination for crystals (urate and pyrophosphate) and culture.
   (ii) blood cultures,
   (iii) X-ray of shoulder.
3. The most likely diagnosis is infective arthritis. Although the most likely causative organism is *Staphylococcus aureus, Streptococci* and Gram negative organisms should also be considered. Initial therapy is empirical until an organism has been isolated and sensitivities are known. A reasonable choice is benzylpenicillin, flucloxacillin, and an aminoglycoside. The joint should be rested and repeatedly aspirated by closed needle drainage until dry. Large joints (e.g. the hip) will need open surgical drainage and this also applies to any joint if there is associated osteomyelitis.
4. Septic arthritis in the elderly is difficult to treat and is associated with a high mortality. There is often slow recovery of function and the development of osteomyelitis.

Discussion

Bacterial arthritis is a common and serious problem in the elderly and approximately 30% of all patients are aged 60 and over. Predisposing factors (present in nearly 65% of elderly with infective arthritis) include those with prosthetic-joints, chronic arthritis (e.g. RA and osteoarthritis) trauma with or without direct puncture wounds, and immunosuppression as a result of an underlying malignancy or steroid therapy. Rheumatoid arthritis is a particularly common predisposing factor and any such patient with a single red painful joint should be considered to have infective arthritis until proven otherwise. *Staphylococcus aureus* is the isolated organism in 80% of rheumatoid infected joints. Gram negative organisms are also commonly found in the elderly.

Further Reading

McGuire, N. M. and Kauffman, C. A., 'Septic arthritis in the elderly' *Journal of the American Geriatrics Society* (1985), **33**, 170–174

Goldberg, D. L. and Reed, J. I., 'Medical progress: Bacterial arthritis', *New England Journal of Medicine* (1985), **312**, 764–771

Case 22

Answers

1. The diagnosis is hydrocephalus of the adult type. It is most likely to be normal or low-pressure hydrocephalus since the patient, in addition to gait disturbance, also has mild intellectual impairment.
2. Insertion of a ventriculo-peritoneal shunt or a ventriculo-atrial shunt. The patients who improve are those who have B waves on recording of CSF pressure. Long-term prognosis however, is poor.

Discussion

Classically, patients with this condition present with the triad of dementia, gait disturbance and incontinence, however, some cases can be asymptomatic and diagnosis made on investigations carried out for unrelated conditions or symptoms.

The aetiology of normal, or low-pressure hydrocephalus is unclear, but incomplete leptomeningeal fibrosis is most common, with or without changes in the arachnoid granules. This may follow trauma or subarachnoid haemorrhage. It is very likely that trauma was the cause in our patient.

Long-term ingestion of barbiturates can lead to a 'dementia' like syndrome.

Further Reading

Briggs, R. S., Castleden, C. M. and Alvarez, A. S., 'Normal pressure hydrocephalus in the elderly: A treatable cause of dementia?' *Age and Ageing* (1981) **10**, 254–258

Pickard, J. D. 'Adult communicating hydrocephalus', *British Journal of Hospital Medicine* (1982), 35–40

Case 23

Answers

1. (i) Postural hypotension secondary to drug therapy and autonomic neuropathy
   (ii) Hyponatraemia due to Moduretic therapy
   (iii) Hypokalaemia due to diuretic therapy
   (iv) Diabetes mellitus
   (v) Urinary tract infection
2. Infusion of saline with potassium and insulin. Antibiotic for infection. Although she required insulin initially, she was taking a oral hypoglycaemic agent (glibenclamide, 5 mg/day) on discharge from hospital.

Discussion

The adverse drug reactions are generally more common in older patients because of their:
(i) greater susceptibility to adverse reactions,
(ii) inadequate diagnosis,

(iii) uncritical assessment of the need for treatment,
(iv) altered pharmacokinetics and sensitivity to drugs and
(v) poor compliance.

This patient did not exhibit the classical symptoms and signs of severe hyponatraemia (i.e. sodium less than 125 mmol/l). In most elderly patients a sodium level of 117 mmol/l will lead to neurological symptoms which may include confusion, muscle twitching, fits and weakness.

Further Reading

'Medication for the elderly', *Drug and Therapeutics* (1984), **22,** 49–52

Arieff, A. I. and Guisado, R., 'Effects on the central nervous system of hypernatraemic and hyponatraemic state', *Kidney International* (1976), **10,** 104–116

Surideram, S. G. and Mankikar, G. D., 'Hyponatraemia in the elderly', *Age and Ageing* (1983), **12,** 77–80

Case 24

Answers

1. (i) Nephrotic syndrome.
   (ii) Diabetes mellitus.
2. Yes: biopsy may reveal changes that are steroid responsive, that is, minimal change.
3. Initial treatment should be with frusemide and spironolactone, with a high protein and low sugar diet. If there is no response and minimal change glomerulonephritis, as in this case, is found on biopsy prednisolone should be added.

Discussion

Nephrotic syndrome, although uncommon, can occur in the elderly. Although membranous nephritis is the commonest finding on biopsy, minimal change is also found in some patients, as illustrated by this case.

The interpretation of renal biopsy specimens are beset with difficulties in the elderly because of age-related changes which affect the glomeruli and blood vessels.

The other renal complications that diabetics may develop include diffuse and nodular glomerulosclerosis, urinary tract infection and, rarely, renal papillary necrosis.

Further Reading

Zech, P., Colon, S., Pointet, P., Deteix, P., Labeeuw, M. and Leitienne, P., 'The nephrotic syndrome in adults aged over 60: etiology, evolution and treatment of 76 cases', *Clinical Nephrology* (1982) **18**, 232–236

Case 25

Answers

1. Intestinal pseudo-obstruction.
2. The chief disorders which can precipitate intestinal pseudo-obstruction are:
   (i) drugs with an atropine-like action,
   (ii) amyloidosis,
   (iii) diabetes mellitus,
   (iv) myxoedema,
   (v) hypoparathyroidism,
   (vi) scleroderma,
   (vii) previous irradiation,
   (viii) heavy metal poisoning,
   (ix) polymyositis and
   (x) varicella
3. Intestinal pseudo-obstruction is an abnormality of intestinal motility producing clinical features of intestinal obstruction. Initial management is aimed at finding a treatable cause. If this cannot be found, management should be aimed at reducing gaseous distension, com-

bating bacterial overgrowth (as abnormal growth of bacteria may contribute to abnormal motility) and stimulating intestinal motility with the use of drugs (e.g. prostigmine). If the colon is dilated by more than 12 cm, it should be decompressed, preferably by a colonoscope. Some patients may also need nasogastric intubation and aspiration with parenteral fluid replacement.

Further Reading

Isaacs, P., Keshavarzian, A., 'Intestinal pseudo-obstruction – a review', *Postgraduate Medical Journal* (1985) **61**, 1033-1038

Case 26

Answers

1. There are many causes of hypokalaemia and all can produce metabolic alkalosis. The increased pigmentation without obvious Cushing's features in this patient suggests the presence of a tumour secreting an ACTH-like hormone. This was confirmed in this patient by elevated serum cortisol (4140 mmol/l (NR 165–700 nmol/l in the morning)) and ACTH levels (705 ng/l (NR 10–80 ng/l)).
   Although there was no need to perform a dexamethazone suppression test, it can be used in difficult cases to distinguish ectopic ACTH production from true Cushing's syndrome. In patients with ectopic ACTH production, suppression is not usually achieved.
2. The aim of management is to correct the metabolic abnormalities and to block the hypothalamo–pituitary–adrenal axis. This patient was given insulin to reduce blood glucose levels, IV fluids and potassium. The pituitary adrenal axis was blocked by metyrapone, a drug which inhibits

the enzyme responsible for 11 β-hydroxylation stage in the synthesis of cortisol.

As this treatment leads to reduced, or no cortisol production, replacement therapy with oral steroids is usually required. In this particular patient the cortisol level fell below 100 nmol/l within 5 days of metyrapone administration (1000 mg qid), despite the addition of prednisolone (5 mg tds). With reduction in metyrapone dosage the cortisol level returned to over 200 nmol/l.

3. To a certain extent this depends upon the patient's wishes, his family's wishes and his social circumstances. His family should be informed about the diagnosis and the prognosis. In view of the poor prognosis, the patient should be referred to a hospice for terminal care if the family or friends are unwilling to provide this at home with community nursing support, and provided the patient is aware of the diagnosis and accepts this plan. If the patient and his family wish to have terminal care at home they can be referred to a community MacMillan nurse, whose interest and experience include terminal care.

Discussion

The causes of hypokalaemia are:
(i) renal – renal tubular acidosis, recovery from obstruction,
(ii) metabolic – aldosteronism, Cushing's disease, ketoacidosis,
(iii) drugs – diuretics, steroids, carbenoxolone, and
(iv) gastrointestinal – vomiting, diarrhoea, purgative abuse, fistulae, villous adenoma, ureterosigmoid anastomasis.

Clinical features of hypokalaemia include non-specific weakness, confusion, paralytic ileus, features of renal tubular damage and conduction defects on ECG.

Further Reading

Rees, L. H., 'The biosynthesis of hormones by non-endocrine tumours – a review', *Journal of Endocrinology* (1975), **67**, 143–175

Case 27

Answers

1. Hypoadrenalism.
2. The recent onset of pigmentation is very significant and highly suggestive of primary hypoadrenalism.
3. (i) Use the long Synacthen test to distinguish between primary and secondary adrenal insufficiency,
   (ii) search for autoantibodies as 63% of those with autoimmune adrenal failure have adrenal antibodies, and
   (iii) perform chest and abdominal X-rays, if adrenal calcification is present it suggests that tuberculosis is the cause of Addison's disease.
4. The drugs which may affect the adrenal cortex include:
   (i) ketoconazole,
   (ii) anticoagulants,
   (iii) etomidate (an anaesthetic agent),
   (iv) excessive alcohol intake (pseudo-Cushing's syndrome),
   (v) metyrapone and aminoglutethimide.
   The last two drugs are used in the management of Cushing's syndrome.

Discussion

Addison's disease, although rare, may be overlooked because of its non-specific features.

Skin pigmentation results from increased levels of ACTH and β-lipotrophin, and is a common early feature of Addison's disease. It should be distinguished from the pigmentation seen with chronic infections, malignancy and chronic renal failure. The pigmentation in Addison's disease occurs on exposed surfaces, skin creases and on areas exposed to pressure from belts and straps. Buccal pigmentation is thought to be due to pressure from the teeth and is often absent in the edentulous elderly.

The commonest causes of primary hypoadrenalism are autoimmune adrenalitis and tuberculosis. Her past history of pernicious anaemia makes the former more likely.

Case 28

Answers

1. (i) Maintain a clear airway; in this case, as the patient is deeply unconscious with depressed reflexes, insert an endotracheal tube and if necessary ventilate artificially.
   (ii) Gastric lavage should be undertaken if the time of overdose is unknown, and absorbers such as activated charcoal, left in the stomach.
   (iii) Give dextrose intravenously, after blood has been taken for blood glucose estimation. Hypoglycaemia is a treatable cause of coma and may be present if alcohol has been taken with the overdosage of tablets.
   (iv) Maintain the circulatory volume. It is, however, important to consider that elderly people are easily pushed into congestive cardiac failure and central venous pressure monitoring may be necessary.
   (v) Monitor renal function.
   (vi) ECG monitoring.
   (vii) Keep the patient warm – elderly people often have impaired thermoregulatory mechanisms and are at risk of hypothermia. This is particularly true of elderly people who have taken barbiturates.
2. Tricyclic or tetracyclic antidepressants are usually the drugs of choice. Repeat overdose attempts can be prevented by giving smaller quantities of drug on discharge, and by regular home visits. In the patient who remains suicidal, agitated or suffers from undue side-effects, electroconvulsive treatment (ECT) may be used.

Discussion

Depression should be managed as aggressively in the elderly as it is in a younger age group. There is usually a good response to initial therapy; however, the long-term prognosis is poor. Only approximately 30% will be well at long-term follow-up. Factors associated with a bad prognosis include depressive delusions, physical ill health and the onset of depression after the age of 70 years.

ECT is usually very effective in the elderly. Memory impairment is minimized if unilateral electrodes are used on the non-dominant side.

Further Reading

Millard, P. H., 'Depression in old age', *British Medical Journal* (1983), **287**, 375–376

Davidson, R., 'The non-drug treatment of depression' (eds. Caird, F. I. and Grimley Evans, I.) *Advanced Geriatric Medicine 3* (1983), Pitman Press, Bath, 119–121

Case 29

Answers

1. Osteomalacia and iron-deficiency anaemia due to malabsorption.
2. Further investigations would include:
   (i) Vitamin B12 and folic acid estimations,
   (ii) bone scanning with or without biopsy to determine the presence of osteomalacia and
   (iii) a jejunal biopsy, ^{14}C glycocholic breath test and culture of jejunal aspirate to detect bacterial overgrowth, measurement of retention of SeHCAT (for malabsorption of bile salts) and an ERCP and ultrasound of the pancreas to determine the cause of malabsorption.
3. Correction of nutrient deficiencies with oral iron and vitamin D. Specific treatment for various conditions producing malabsorption may be helpful in patients with coeliac disease or in those with bacterial overgrowth. In coeliac disease a gluten-free diet may be useful if diarrhoea and abdominal pain are prominent symptoms. With bacterial overgrowth, antibiotics such as tetracycline or cotrimoxazole have been found to be beneficial.

Discussion

Although there is a decline with age in intake of all nutrients, clinical malnutrition is rare, perhaps affecting 1–2% of elderly in the community. This is likely to occur in those who have physical and mental disabilities and those who are depressed, apathetic or recently bereaved and those who live alone or in long-stay institutions.

SeHCAT is a synthetic bile salt containing selenium-75, which can be used to detect malabsorption of bile acid.

Further Reading

Badenoch, J., 'Steatorrhoea in the adult', *British Medical Journal* (1960), **ii**, 880

Merrick, M. V., Eastwood, M. A. and Ford, M. J. 'Is bile acid malabsorption underdiagnosed? An evaluation of accuracy of diagnosis of measurement of SeHCAT retention', *British Medical Journal* (1985), **290**, 665–668

Case 30

Answers

1. Raised intracranial pressure.
2. (i) Cerebral tumour,
   (ii) cerebral abscess.
3. CT scan of the brain. In this particular patient a mass in the right frontoparietal region was demonstrated, and subsequent biopsy revealed a malignant glioma.

Discussion

This lady has 2 cardinal features of raised intracranial pressure: those of headache and progressive drowsiness (other features of raised intracranial pressure in the elderly are apathy, increasing immobility, confusion and progressive focal cerebral disorder). The characteristics of the headache in this patient are rather atypical, but disease does not always conform to the text book description. In addition, in the elderly, history may be inaccurate, particularly in the presence of cognitive impairment, which is suggested in this case by the recent onset of memory impairment.

The absence of papilloedema does not exclude raised intracranial pressure and patients can die from rapidly increasing intracranial pressure without ever developing papilloedema. Skull X-rays are of little value and if there is deteriorating level of consciousness, an urgent CT scan should be requested.

The differential diagnosis of headache includes a raised intracranial pressure due to a space-occupying lesion, temporal arteritis, meningitis, referred pain from the teeth, cervical spine or chest, sinusitis, middle-ear disease, glaucoma, viral illness, tension headache, trigeminal neuralgia and drugs (e.g. vasodilators, calcium antagonists).

Further Reading

Twomey, C., 'Brain tumours in the elderly', *Age and Ageing* (1978), **7**, 138–145

Case 31

Answers

1. The probable diagnosis is scleroderma.
2. (i) Evidence of vasculitis,
   (ii) Raynaud's phenomenon,
   (iii) depigmentation or hyperpigmentation,
   (iv) telangiectasia,
   (v) sclerodactyly,
   (vi) subcutaneous calcification and
   (vii) features of Sjögren's (Sicca) syndrome.

3. The most commonly involved system is the gastrointestinal tract with oesophageal involvement in up to 90% of cases.
4. The treatment is difficult and unsatisfactory. Improvements have, however, been noted with D-penicillamine, colchicine and steroids. Hypertension associated with this condition responds well to ACE inhibitors and there is a suggestion that captopril modifies the disease.

   If there is synovitis anti-inflammatory drugs should be tried. The medical treatment of other complications includes metoclopramide administration to improve oesophageal motility, antibiotic administration for bacterial overgrowth in the gastrointestinal tract.

Discussion

Scleroderma is a multisystem disease. Renal involvement (although uncommon in the elderly) is indicated by abnormal urinary sediment, proteinuria and hypertension. Pulmonary involvement may be indicated by pleuritic disease, pulmonary hypertension or pulmonary interstitial fibrosis. The CREST syndrome consists of Calcinosis, Raynaud's phenomenom, Oesophageal involvement, Sclerodactyly and Telangiectasia

Sjögren's syndrome – This is characterized by infiltration of exocrine glands and other organs by plasma cells and lymphocytes. The major clinical features are dryness of the eyes and mouth. The former can lead to desiccation of the cornea and conjunctiva, corneal ulceration or perforation. Systemic involvement is variable but can lead to diffuse interstitial pneumonitis, renal tubular defects, cranial nerve involvement and non-thrombocytopenic purpura. This syndrome can present in patients with scleroderma (rarely) as well as those with rheumatoid arthritis, SLE or biliary cirrhosis. Diagnoses are usually made on clinical grounds but can be confirmed by Schirmer's test or lip biopsy.

Further Reading

Bellamy, N., Kean, W. E. and Buchanan, W. W., 'Connective tissue diseases', *Hospital Update* (1984), **10**, 135–146

Case 32

Answers

1. Pituitary adenoma. Although most adenomas are thought to be non-secretory over 50% contain prolactin-secreting cells.
2. (i) A visual field test by clinical confrontation as well as perimetry, to detect evidence of any local effect.
   (ii) Endocrine investigations to detect hypopituitarism (i.e. levels of prolactin FSH and LH and thyroid function tests including the TRH test and the adrenal axis).
   (iii) CT scan.
3. In view of her general state, radiotherapy was recommended in addition to giving her hydrocortisone for her hypoadrenalism (found on investigation).

Discussion

Pituitary tumours can be asymptomatic and discovered only when investigations are carried out for either cerebrovascular disease or confusion. Symptomatic tumours may present with signs and symptoms due to pressure on local structures or with alterations in the secretion of hormones. Local effects not only lead to headaches but visual disturbances, nerve palsies (third, fourth, sixth and all olfactory nerves), the hypothalamic syndrome (e.g. increased appetite or diabetes insipidus) or CSF rhinorrhoea. Hormonal changes are usually those of hypopituitarism. In case of ACTH deficiency, patients may complain of vomiting, falls or symptoms of hypoglycaemia.

Asymptomatic patients without any pressure effects or endocrine abnormalities require no treatment but observation.

Symptomatic tumours should be treated with surgery. If, however, the patient is not fit for surgery then yttrium rod implantation or radiotherapy should be considered. Those elderly with tumours and oversecretion of growth hormone may also benefit from the use of bromocriptine.

Further Reading

Murphy, P. J. and Rai, G. S., 'Pituitary tumours – an increasing incidence', *Geriatric Medicine* (1984), **14,** 181–183

Case 33

Answers

1. (i) Faecal impaction.
   (ii) Urinary tract infection.
   (iii) Breast carcinoma.
   (iv) Confusional state secondary to dementia. The latter was confirmed in our patient by the long history of confusion and memory loss.
   (v) Spondylolisthesis at L4/5.
   (vi) Peripheral vascular disease.
2. Initial management should be treatment of impaction (with enemas and lactulose) and the urinary tract infection with ampicillin.
3. In view of the patient's age and mental state, it would be advisable to treat this medically with tamoxifen (which has an anti-oestrogen action) provided that her daughter takes on the responsibility to give her the drug. If then the lump begins to ulcerate local irradiation should be considered.
4. There is no single treatment that will increase the bone mass in this woman; available treatment may only prevent or slow down the bone loss. However, in view of this woman's mental state and the likelihood of poor compliance, no treatment should be given particularly since she has no symptoms at the present time.

Discussion

Faecal incontinence is a very common symptom which can be produced by:
(i) impaction of faeces,

(ii) carcinoma of rectum,
(iii) rectal prolapse,
(iv) inflammatory bowel disease,
(v) villous adenoma,
(vi) previous surgical operation on the ano-rectum,
(vii) incompetence of the sphincter,
(viii) pelvic floor neuropathy and
(ix) dementia.

Management is aimed at identifying the cause and treating it. If this does not help, then it may be assumed that patient is suffering from neurogenic incontinence. These patients may be helped by alternating courses of constipating agent and a mild laxative. Some patients with sphincter problems also benefit from surgical treatment such as sphincter reconstruction.

Tamoxifen which has anti-oestrogen actions can produce a beneficial effect, not only in patients who have oestrogen receptor positive tumour but also in those in whom no oestrogen receptors are detected.

Case 34

Answers

1. (i) Hypoglycaemia.
   (ii) Pneumonia in a patient with chronic airflow obstruction and pulmonary hypertension.
   (iii) Chronic renal failure.
2. (i) Excess alcohol intake.
   (ii) Malnutrition.
   (iii) Septicaemia from pneumonia.
3. Intravenous glucose and antibiotics.

Discussion

The common causes of hypoglycaemia are excess insulin and long-acting sulphonylureas in diabetic patients and the presence of insulin secreting tumours. The former can result because of incorrect dosage of insulin or sulphonylureas or omission of meals. Initial symptoms of sweating, shaking and palpitations may not be marked in the elderly, who may present with confusion, drowsiness or stroke. chronic hypoglycaemia may lead to dementia.

All sulphonylureas, even tolbutamide and glibenclamide, can lead to hypoglycaemia despite their stated short half-life. However, in the elderly requiring hypoglycaemic therapy tolbutamide is the drug of choice.

Further Reading

Gale, E., 'Causes of hypoglycaemia', *British Journal of Hospital Medicine* (1985), **33**, 159–162

Case 35

Answers

1. The causes of haematuria include:
   - (i) renal tract tumours, calculi, infection and trauma,
   - (ii) prostatic hypertrophy in men,
   - (iii) systemic diseases including blood dyscrasias and blood clotting defects,
   - (iv) primary renal diseases like nephritis, infarction or renal vein thrombosis,
   - (v) side-effects of anticoagulation and
   - (vi) A–V malformations.
2. Investigations which this patient should undergo include:
   - (i) urine culture with early morning specimen for culture of AFBs,
   - (ii) microscopy for casts to exclude nephritis,
   - (iii) coagulation screen,
   - (iv) ultrasound and or IVP followed by cystoscopy and retrograde pyelogram, or both.
3. Yes. Ultrasound is a very sensitive screening test for a renal mass.

Discussion

Infection and tumour are the 2 common causes of haematuria in clinical practice; therefore, any elderly patient presenting with haematuria without urinary tract infection should be investigated fully.

Further Reading

Clayman, R. V., Surya, V., Miller, R. P., Reinke, D. B. and Fraley, E. F., 'Pursuit of the renal mass: is ultrasound enough?', *American Journal of Medicine* (1984), **77**, 218–223

Case 36

Answers

1. (i) Degenerative joint disease.
   (ii) Cardiac arrythmias secondary to drug therapy or myocardial ischaemia.
   (iii) Hypotension following myocardial ischaemia or secondary drug therapy.
   (iv) Poor vision.
   (v) Proximal muscle weakness secondary to osteomalacia. (The presence of osteomalacia is suggested by the biochemical changes.)
   (vi) Parkinson's disease with associated gait abnormalities.
2. (i) Dementia.
   (ii) Failure of treatment resulting in 'on and off' phenomenon and 'freezing' episodes.
3. Terminate Artane therapy since the incidence of side-effects with anticholinergic drugs is high; these drugs may also contribute to intellectual impairment. In addition, Sinemet dosage should be titrated against patient response. The patient may have to be given Sinemet 3–4 hourly to achieve the maximum effect.

Discussion

The characteristic Parkinsonian tremor is often absent in the elderly. The other symptoms of Parkinson's disease such as difficulty in walking, getting in and out of bed or problems with dressing tend to be labelled in early stages of the disease as being due to old age; this may lead to a late diagnosis of the condition.

In addition to drug therapy, elderly patients with Parkinson's disease benefit from assessment and treatment from physiotherapists, speech therapists and occupational therapists, particularly when the drugs start to lose their effect. Physiotherapists may not only be able to improve balance and walking but may be able to teach so called 'trick movements' to overcome 'freezing'.

Atrial tachycardia with AV block can result from an ectopic focus or re-entry via aberrant pathway. During the attack there may be polyurea due to the elaboration of natriuretic peptide by the atrial tissue.

Further Reading

Hardie, R., 'Treatment of Parkinson's disease', *British Journal of Hospital Medicine* (1985), **33**, 45

Case 37

Answers

1. The increased uptake by the spleen in the presence of patchy or poor uptake by the liver suggests hepatic cell dysfunction. The degree of uptake by spleen reflects the degree of hepatic damage.
2. Peripheral neuropathy probably due to alcohol.
3. Depression, falls leading to rib fractures, dehydration, mild confusion, bruising, anorexia and distended abdomen.

Discussion

In normal ageing there are distal sensory impairment and depression or loss of distal reflexes as a result of distal axonal degeneration but patients tend not to have any symptoms.

Chronic polyneuropathy of old age is a relatively benign condition which leads to symptoms involving the lower limbs and although the predominant features are sensory, in some it can lead to foot drop.

With alcoholism in the elderly there is often no history available. Some seem to have a stable working life and only develop overt alcoholic problems after retirement. Possible factors include bereavement, social withdrawal and changes of ageing. Once liver disease has developed the prognosis is very poor with 48% dying within 1 year of presentation.

Further Reading

Desai, H. N. and Arunachalam, S., 'When age plus alcoholism can be misleading', *Geriatric Medicine* (1980), **10,** 11–14

Olney, R., 'Age-related changes in peripheral nerve function' *Geriatric Medicine Today* (1985) **4,** 76–86

Woodhouse, K. W. and James, O. F. W., 'Alcoholic liver, disease in the elderly. Presentation and outcome', *Age and Ageing* (1985), **14,** 113–118

Case 38

Answers

1. (i) Non-ketotic hyperosmolar coma,
   (ii) bronchopneumonia,
   (iii) recent anterior myocardial infarction.
2. The probable precipitating factors in this case include infection, myocardial infarction and thiazide diuretic.
3. This is a medical emergency and the treatment should consist of correction of fluid and electrolyte abnormalities, administration of insulin and treatment of any underlying

causes. The choice of fluid replacement remains controversial; however the majority favour replacement with 50% normal saline solution and aim to correct the fluid deficit in at least 48 hours. This should avoid rapid changes in osmolality and thus worsening of cerebral function. Insulin is the mainstay of treatment and is usually given by intravenous infusion. As there is a clinical evidence of bronchopneumonia, this patient should be given an antibiotic.

4. The prognosis is poor. There is a high mortality associated with this condition and the quoted figures vary from 20–50%

Discussion

This syndrome usually occurs in the elderly and the majority are known diabetic patients. However, it can occur in nondiabetic patients as a complication of extensive burns, heat stroke, acute pancreatitis, infections, surgery, thyrotoxicosis, acromegaly, dialysis, and with use of certain drugs (e.g. diuretics steroids, phenytoin and propanolol).

As a group the elderly are susceptible to dehydration probably as a result of the age-related changes of reduced sensation to thirst and blunted renal response to ADH in the presence of reduced renal concentrating ability.

Further Reading

Khardori, R. and Soler, N. G., 'Hyperosmolar hyperglycaemic non-ketotic syndrome: Report of 22 cases and brief review', *American Journal of Medicine* (1984), **77**, 899–904

Case 39

Answers

1. (i) Subacute bacterial endocarditis.
   (ii) Congestive heart failure.
   (iii) Iron-deficiency anaemia.
   (iv) Right hemiparesis secondary to embolus resulting from subacute bacterial endocarditis.

(v) Gout.
2. Large left atrium.
3. (i) Diuretic for heart failure. In this patient captopril was added as the patient showed no improvement on diuretic therapy alone.
(ii) Benzyl penicillin with probenecid until the culture comes back positive. Treatment should be continued for at least 3 weeks.
(iii) Iron therapy for iron-deficiency anaemia.
(iv) Azapropazone or indomethacin or colchicine for acute gout.

Discussion

The frequency of infective endocarditis in the older population is increasing. As in other infections it can present with only non-specific symptoms in patients with no valvular disease; therefore the clinical index of suspicion needs to be high. A heart murmur in the elderly person should not be discarded as simply being due to degenerative valve disease. The commonest organism is *Streptococcus viridans* but any organism including *Diphtheroids* and *Candida* can produce endocarditis.

Prognosis is usually very poor but this is thought to reflect delay in diagnosis and initiation of treatment.

Further Reading

Oakley, C. M., 'Infective endocarditis' *British Journal of Hospital Medicine* (1980), **24,** 232–243

Schnurr, L. R., Ball, A. P., Geddes, A. M., Gray, J. and McGhie, D., 'Bacterial endocarditis in England in the 1970s: a review of 70 patients', *Quarterly Journal of Medicine (NS)* (1977), **46,** 499–512

Case 40

Answers

1. Thiazide diuretics, vitamin D and lithium are the important drugs to enquire about in patients with hypercalcaemia.

2. Important initial investigations include:
   (i) repeating the serum calcium in a fasting state without the use of tourniquet to verify the raised calcium,
   (ii) a full blood count,
   (iii) ESR,
   (iv) an estimation of serum phosphate, alkaline phosphatase, urea, creatinine, serum chloride, serum bicarbonate, serum thyroxine blood levels,
   (v) X-rays of the hands and chest and
   (vi) an estimation of PTH levels.
3. The 2 most likely diagnoses are malignancy and primary hyperparathyroidism. These account for 92% of all cases of hypercalcaemia in hospital.
4. The postulated mechanisms include:
   (i) peptide with PTH-like action produced by the tumour,
   (ii) extensive bony metastases,
   (iii) prostaglandins,
   (iv) growth promoting factor and
   (v) osteoclast activating factor.

Discussion

The tests which can be used in distinguishing primary hyperparathyroidism from other causes of hypercalcaemia include the steroid suppression test and multivariate analysis. A significant suppression on steroid is a fall in serum calcium of >0.25 mmol/l and this by and large indicates that hypercalcaemia is due to cause(s) other than primary hyperparathyroidism.

Hyperparathyroidism is common and has an incidence of 26 per 250 000 population. It is now a disease of the middle-aged and elderly female. The presentation has also changed over the years with the hypercalcaemia being an incidental finding. The management of these asymptomatic patients is, at present, unsettled due to uncertainty about the natural history of the condition.

Multivariate analysis is based on deriving discriminant functions using serum phosphate, alkaline phosphatase, albumin, globulin and potassium to assist in classification of the more difficult cases of hypercalcaemia (Grero and Hodkinson, 1977) The discriminant function is the sum of test values each multiplied by a weighting factor derived from analysis of previous cases in order to obtain maximum separation of the distribution of function between the various conditions producing hypercalcaemia.

Further Reading

Fisken, R. A., Heath, D. A. and Bold, A. M., 'Hypercalcaemia – a hospital survey', *Quarterly Journal of Medicine* (1980), **49**, 405–418

Grero, P. S. and Hodkinson, H. M., 'Hypercalcaemia in elderly hospital patients: value of discriminant analysis in differential diagnosis.' *Age and Ageing* (1977), **6**, 14–20

Stevenson, J. C., 'Editorial: Malignant hypercalcaemia', *British Medical Journal* (1986), **291**, 421–422

Scholz, D. A. and Purnell, D. C., 'Asymptomatic primary hyperparathyroidism', *Mayo Clinic Proceedings* (1981), **56**, 473–478

Case 41

Answers

1. This patient has myelodysplastic anaemia (as indicated by bone marrow appearance) and no response to therapy with B12 and folic acid.
2. There is no specific treatment for this condition. The course is usually a chronic one and some require repeated blood transfusions.
3. The 5 causes of macrocytosis can be any of the following:
   (i) liver disease,
   (ii) chronic alcoholism,
   (iii) haemolytic anaemia,
   (iv) haemorrhage,
   (v) multiple myeloma,
   (vi) Waldenstrom's macroglobinaemia,
   (vii) hypothyroidism,
   (viii) chronic obstructive airways disease,
   (ix) primary sideroblastic anaemia,
   (x) acquired sideroblastic anaemia.

(xi) aplastic anaemia,
(xii) leucoerythroblastic anaemia,
(xiii) anti-convulsant therapy and
(xiv) cytotoxic therapy.

Discussion

Myelodysplastic syndromes are characteristically found in the elderly, usually as anaemias refractory to haematinic replacement. They may have associated neutropenia and thrombocytopenia, , or both. Gross enlargement of the liver, spleen and lymph nodes is not found, although mild enlargement of the spleen may occur in 5% to 30% of patients. The bone marrow is hypercellular with morphological abnormalities in all cell lines. The clinical course is chronic and variable and some patients require repeated blood transfusions. The survival range is from a few months to as long as 10 to 15 years. Death usually results from complications of neutropenia and thrombocytopenia, or both, and in some it terminates in an acute leukaemic state.

Despite the haemoglobin levels of 8.6 g/dl this patient had no symptoms of anaemia.

Further Reading

McLennan, W. J., Andrews, G. R., MacLeod, C. and Caird, F. I., 'Anaemia in the elderly', *Quarterly Journal of Medicine (NS)* (1973), **XLII,** 1–13

Antin, J. H. and Rosenthal, D. S., 'Acute leukaemia, myelodysplasia and lymphoma', Freedman, M. L. (ed.) *'Clinics in Geriatric Medicine',* W. B. Saunders Company, Philadelphia, London (1985), **1,** (4), 795–826

Case 42

Answers

1. (i) Right lower lobe pneumonia.
   (ii) Hiatus hernia.

(iii) Volvulus of stomach.
(iv) Tetraparesis due to cerebral palsy.

2. Volvulus of stomach.
3. Complications of volvulus of stomach are fluid and electrolyte loss and strangulation.

   Treatment is surgery in patients with acute volvulus or with recurrent chronic volvulus. Operations which have been found to be useful include repair of diaphragmatic hernia, gastropexy and repair of eventration of the diaphragm.

   In some the volvulus may be corrected by decompression using a nasogastric tube; however, it is recognized that failure to pass the nasogastric tube is one of the features of gastric volvulus.
4. (i) Achalasia.
   (ii) Oesophageal spasm.

Discussion

Two of the well known causes of dysphagia in the elderly are achalasia and diffuse oesophageal spasm.

In achalasia the treatment is dilatation or cardiomyectomy, but in those who are unfit or unwilling to have surgery relief can be given using isosorbide dinitrate sublingually before meals.

In oesophageal spasm the symptoms are intermittent consisting of dysphagia and retrosternal chest pain which might resemble cardiac pain. Diagnosis can be made on manometric studies or radiology. If symptoms are severe the patient can be given isosorbide or nifedipine sublingually.

Aspiration pneumonia is a common problem in frail elderly people. The contributing factors of this condition include:

(i) deterioration of cough, pharyngeal and laryngeal reflexes with age,
(ii) neurological disorders that depress consciousness or affect the above mentioned reflexes and
(iii) oesophageal disorders.

The type and severity of pulmonary reaction depends upon the quantity of aspirate. Highly acid gastric content, can lead to pneumonia which resembles respiratory distress syndrome.

Further Reading

Wastell, C. and Ellis, H., 'Volvulus of the stomach: a review with report of 8 cases', *British Journal of Surgery*, (1971), **58**, 557–562.
'Editorial: Dysphagia in the elderly', *Journal of the American Geriatric Society*, (1986), **34**, 248–249

Case 43

Answers

1. In view of the symptom of burning when swallowing hot liquids the most likely diagnosis is oesophagitis (cf. Bernstein's test). The causes include:
   (i) peptic oesophagitis due to reflux,
   (ii) local irritant effects of potassium chloride tablets secondary to hold-up,
   (iii) scleroderma or Barrett's oesophagus,
   (iv) candidiasis,
   (v) obstructive lesions (e.g. carcinoma),
   (vi) systemic disorders such as Crohn's disease or Behcet's disease and
   (vii) oesophageal motility disorders (e.g. achalasia).
2. Yes. Drugs are well-known causes of oesophagitis. The drugs which can produce this effect include antibiotics, emepronium bromide, potassium chloride tablets (Slow K), non-steroidal anti-inflammatory drugs and ferrous sulphate.
3. The investigations which should be carried out include:
   (i) barium meal and endoscopy to delineate any structural lesion and
   (ii) a screen for motility disorders if the endoscopy and barium meal reveal no abnormal features. The diagnosis in this patient was candidiasis of the oesophagus.

Discussion

Candidiasis is the most common fungal infection of the gastrointestinal tract. Involvement of the oesophagus is likely to occur in immunosuppressed patients (especially in those with lymphoid, haematological and solid tumour malignancies), in those with oesophageal carcinoma, in those with endocrine disorders (e.g. hypoparathyroidism, hypothyroidism, adrenal insufficiency and diabetes mellitus) and in those with poor nutrition. Symptoms include dysphagia especially when eating solids, retrosternal pain or bleeding. Oral thrush may be found in 50% of patients with oesophageal candidiasis.

Although dysphagia may be the presenting symptom of oesophageal candidiasis, nearly 50% are asymptomatic.

Further Reading

Kikendal, J. W., Friedman, A. C., Oyewole, M. A., Fleischer, D. and Johnson, L. S., 'Pill-induced oesophageal injury: case reports and review of the medical literature', *Digestive Diseases and Sciences* (1983), **28**, 174–182

Trier, J. S. and Bjorkman, D. J. 'Oesophageal, gastric and intestinal candidiasis', *American Journal of Medicine* (1984), **77** (4D), 39–43

Case 44

Answers

1. (i) Phimosis leading to hydronephrosis and chronic renal failure.
   (ii) Dehydration leading to acute or chronic renal failure and hypernatraemia.
   (iii) Probable septicaemia from urinary tract infection.
   (iv) Mild anaemia due to chronic renal failure with or without concomitant malnutrition.
2. (i) Rehydration with 5% dextrose with careful monitoring of sodium, potassium and urine flows.
   (ii) Antibiotics.
   (iii) A suprapubic catheter had to be introduced in the patient as a temporary measure prior to circumcision.

3. The future plan will depend on patient's recovery from his acute illnesses, his physical and mental state at the time and on his wishes. However, as the patient was living in squalid conditions and was unable to cope his discharge should be delayed until:
   (i) the flat is cleaned up and
   (ii) a home visit is carried out to assess his capabilities and needs for services and alterations to the flat.

   If the outcome of the home visit is positive then the patient's discharge should be organized with the services indicated by the home visit. If however, the patient would always require some degree of supervision, he should be approached and given the various choices of habitation that are available in the district; these may include not only warden-controlled flats or Part III accommodation but also adult fostering arrangements which are available in some parts of the country. Depending upon his wishes appropriate application should be made.

Discussion

The symptoms of hypernatraemia are often non-specific in the early stages. Symptoms which the patient usually complains of vary from weakness to drowsiness to coma, muscle rigidity and fits.

Further Reading

Bay, W. H. and Ferris, T. F., 'Hypernatraemia and hyponatraemia Disorders of toxicity', *Geriatrics* (1976), **31**, 53–64

Case 45

Answers

1. The association of hyponatraemia and low plasma osmolality suggest inappropriate ADH secretion secondary to either hypothyroidism or head injury.

2. (i) An ECG

   Long-standing hypothyroidism is associated with a considerable degree of atherosclerosis. A normal ECG does not exclude ischaemic heart disease but an abnormal ECG would suggest that extreme caution was needed in initiating replacement therapy.

   (ii) The short Synacthen test

   With this degree of hyponatraemia it is important to exclude hypoadrenalism because, if this coexists with hypothyroidism, treatment of the latter could precipitate an Addisonian crisis.

3. If there is no evidence of ischaemic heart disease, thyroxine replacement therapy should commence with no more than 0.025 mg thyroxine daily. This should be increased by monthly increments of 0.025 mg thyroxine until the correct replacement dose is obtained.

   In the presence of symptomatic ischaemic heart disease one must be even more cautious and if there are no contra-indications to beta blockade this may provide myocardial protection. There is no advantage in using tri-iodothyronine (T3).

4. (i) Hypothermia.

   (ii) Beta-blockade.

Discussion

The commonest cause of hypothyroidism in the elderly is autoimmune thyroiditis. The prevalence increases with age, and is 0.5% in women over the age of 65 years.

The diagnosis is often overlooked in the elderly because of its insidious onset and non-specific symptoms which are often attributed to ageing alone. The classical picture is rarely seen however, since approximately 70% of patients are thought to present atypically.

A low T4 is not diagnostic as this is also seen in the 'sick euthyroid syndrome'. A diagnosis of primary hypothyroidism must be supported by a raised TSH concentration.

Anaemia may result from coexisting pernicious anaemia or as a direct effect of hypothyroidism (probably mediated via decreased erythropoietin levels). Macrocytosis is commonly seen; indeed even after excluding pernicious anaemia 41% of elderly hypothyroid patients are macrocytic compared to 9% euthyroid age-matched controls.

Further Reading

Tunbridge, W. M., Evered, D. G., Hall, R., Appleton, D., Brewis, M., Clark, F., Evans, J. G., Young, E., Bird, T. and Smith, P. A., 'The specturm of thyroid disease in a community: the Wickham survey', *Clinical Endocrinology* (1977), **7**, 481–493

Case 46

Answers

1. Cardiac arrhythmias.
2. In view of the R on T phenomenon she should be given anti-arrhythmic therapy as a significant number of patients with this phenomenon go on to develop ventricular tachycardia. In this woman disopyramide was given in an initial dose of 100 mg bd which was later increased to 100 mg tds.
3. In the majority of cases, urinary incontinence can be caused by simple factors like urinary tract infection, confusion, poor mobility, atrophic vaginitis, constipation, vaginal prolapse, the use of drugs such as loop diuretics and bladder instability. Most of these can be excluded by history, examination and simple investigation. It is unnecessary to refer every patient for invasive tests in the urodynamic clinic. In this patient, the factors responsible for her incontinence were confusion, poor mobility and impaction, although rectal examination was normal. Impaction was confirmed on plain abdominal X-ray film.
4. The patient's relatives should be informed that the confusion results from acute medical problems and that the prognosis is good.

Discussion

Apart from simple causes, incontinence in the elderly can be due to an unstable bladder, stress incontinence due to pelvic floor damage and retention with overflow as seen in enlarged prostate or impaction of faeces or vaginal prolapse.

The unstable bladder can be treated with bladder training and drugs like imipramine or oxybutynin chloride. Stress incontinence can be improved in some patients with pelvic exercises. Patients with retention with overflow need removal of the obstruction and in those who have large residual urine, repeated catheterizations may be helpful. Incontinence is present in 11.6% of women and 6.7% of men over the age of 65 years.

Patients with acute confusional state are often labelled as suffering from dementia which is a chronic, progressive and irreversible condition. The important distinguishing features of the acute confusional state are:

(i) the abrupt onset of confusion,
(ii) the presence of restlessness and anxiety with or without hallucinations,
(iii) the fluctuation of the degree of symptoms with the patient's lucid intervals,
(iv) the presence of delusions in interpretation of external events and surroundings,
(v) the reversible nature of the condition (often resulting from a physical disease) when appropriately treated, and
(vi) the patient's intellect is often still good.

Further Reading

Thomas, T. M., Plymat, K. R., Blannin, J. and Meade, J. W., 'Prevalance of urinary incontinence', *British Medical Journal* (1980), **281**, 1243–1245

Case 47

Answers

1. This man has increased free T4 and T3 levels and is therefore thyrotoxic.
2. This patient should be initially rendered euthyroid using an antithyroid drug such as carbimazole (45 mg per day).

The concurrent use of beta blockers is often advocated but they are of little value and may be dangerous in the elderly except in those with thyrotoxid crisis. Beta blockers should certainly be avoided in the elderly with heart failure.

Once euthyroid, radioactive iodine is usually the treatment of choice in the elderly.

3. (i) Cholestasis.
   (ii) Congestive cardiac failure.
   (iii) Thyrotoxicosis.

Discussion

Thyrotoxicosis in the elderly often presents atypically. Ocular manifestations are rare and symptoms may be few. Symptoms and signs if present are often referred to one system, usually the cardiovascular system, suggesting primary disease of the heart.

'Apathetic thyrotoxicosis' is common in the elderly. It is usually associated with a long history of apathy and anorexia with considerable weight loss and is easily misdiagnosed as depression.

The interpretation of thyroid function tests can be difficult in the presence of another acute illness. However, whereas free thyroxine levels may be low, normal or elevated in 'sick euthyroid' syndrome, T3 levels are invariably low. In the early stages of thyrotoxicosis or in the presence of an autonomous nodule an elevated T3 may be the only biochemical abnormality.

Certain drugs can interfere with thyroid function tests. These include oestrogens, androgens, salicylates, phenytoin, phenylbutazone, fenclofenac, beta blockers and amiodarone. Fenclofenac competitively inhibits the binding of thyroxine (T4) and tri-iodothyronine (T3) to the thyroid binding proteins leading to decreased hormone levels. Amiodarone inhibits peripheral conversion of T4 to T3; this is characterized by increased serum but decreased T3.

Further Reading

Thomas, F. B., Mazzaferri, E. L. and Skillman, T. G., 'Apathetic thyrotoxicosis: a distinctive clinical and laboratory entity',

Annals of Internal Medicine (1970), **72**, 679–685
Morley, J. E., Slag, M. E., Elson, M. K. and Shafer, R. B., 'The interpretation of thyroid function tests in hospitalised patients', *Journal of the American Medical Association* (1983), **249**, 2377–2379

Case 48

Answers

1. Waldenstrom's macroglobulinaemia, hyperviscosity syndrome and focal neurological disturbance.
2. (i) Plasmaphaeresis to decrease viscosity of blood.
   (ii) Cytotoxic drugs (e.g. cyclophosphamide, melphalan or chlorambucil with or without steroids).
3. Prognosis is generally good provided complications are treated as they occur. The median survival in those who respond to chemotherapy is 49 months and in non-responders the median survival is 24 months.
4. In view of the changes in her social and personal circumstances (i.e. death of her husband and loss of confidence in herself) she will require repeated reassurances from the multi-disciplinary team, a home visit prior to discharge and possible counselling for a grief reaction.

Discussion

Waldenstrom's macroglobulinaemia is a disease of elderly with the average age of the patient being 60 years. Two thirds of the patients are males, and the hallmark of the condition is the presence of a monoclonal IgM paraprotein produced by a clone of immature B lymphocytes. Clinical symptoms include fatigue, weakness, haemorrhages, weight loss, neurological disturbances, visual disturbances and Raynaud's phenomenon. Neurological disturbances that may occur not only include cerebral dysfunction and confusion but polyneuritis or polyreticulitis associated with increase in spinal fluid protein.

Physical findings include hepatomegaly in 38% of patients, splenomegaly in 37%, ocular changes in 37%, lymphadenopathy in 37%, haematological abnormalities in approximately 20%, purpura in 17% and congestive cardiac failure in about 4%.

A closely related entity which is benign and occurs in the elderly is benign monoclonal gammopathy. This was also described by Waldenstrom. In this the level of IgG does not exceed 2 g/l and the level of other immunoglobins are not depressed. Plasma cells in the bone marrow do not exceed 9% and there is no Bence-Jones proteinuria.

Further Reading

Denel, T. F., Davis, P. and Avioli, L. V., 'Waldenstrom's macroglobulinaemia', *Archives of Internal Medicine* (1983), **143,** 986–988

'Editorial: Waldenstrom's macroglobulinaemia', *Lancet* (1985), **ii,** 311–312

Kyle, R. A. and Greipp, P. R., 'The laboratory investigation of monoclonal gammopathies', *Mayo Clinic Proceedings* (1978), **53,** 719–739

Case 49

Answers

1. Rapid rewarming was not indicated in this case. Rapid surface rewarming is associated with skin vasodilatation with an accompanying fall in core temperature and circulatory collapse.
2. Resistant hypothermia is associated with hypothyroidism, hypoadrenalism, hypothalamic lesions, head injuries, Wernicke's encephalopathy and treatment with drugs such as phenothiazines and barbiturates.
3. (i) Inappropriate ADH secretion due to hypothyroidism or pneumonia.
   (ii) Secondary to diuretic therapy.
   (iii) Hypoadrenalism.
4. (i) TSH measurement.
   (ii) TRH test (if TSH is normal) to exclude secondary hypothroidism.
   (iii) Synacthen test.

Discussion

Elderly hypothermic patients with a deep body temperature greater than 32°C should be rewarmed at a rate of 0.5°C per hour to avoid circulatory collapse.

Initial rapid core rewarming is indicated if the rectal temperature is less than 28°C or if the patient has uncontrollable diabetes mellitus, since insulin has little or no effect at low temperatures.

Ventricular fibrillation and asystole are likely to occur at rectal temperatures less than 32.2°C and the former is particularly resistant to treatment at these low temperatures.

The measurement of total T4 is of little value in acutely ill people. Abnormalities of total T4 and free T4 and T3 are frequently seen even when the patient is euthyroid. However, in the 'sick euthyroid' syndrome TSH levels are nearly always normal, thus distinguishing it from primary hypothyroidism.

If pituitary function is normal it is important to exclude hypoadrenalism since, if this coexists with hypothyroidism, treatment of the latter may precipitate an Addisonian crisis.

Further Reading

Hyams, D. E., 'Hypothermic myxoedema coma', *British Journal of Clinical Practice* (1963), **17**, 1–14

Maclean, D., Griffiths, D., Browning, M. C. and Murison, J., 'Metabolic aspects of spontaneous rewarming', *Quarterly Journal of Medicine* (1974), **43**, 371–387

Emslie-Smith, D., 'Hypothermia in the elderly', *British Journal of Hospital Medicine* (1981), **26**, 442–450

Case 50

Answers

1. Gas under the diaphragm from perforation of peptic ulcer.
2. (i) Stop indomethacin as there is no real indication for

its use. Risks associated with NSAID have now been highlighted by many studies and these include not only gastrointestinal bleeding but adverse renal and electrolyte disturbances.
   (ii) Start cimetidine therapy.
3. No treatment presently available increases bone mass and strength in osteoporosis once the fracture has occurred. Therapies that have been tried singly and in combination in the younger elderly patients which have been found to prevent further bone loss include:
   (i) oestrogens,
   (ii) calcium supplements,
   (iii) fluoride,
   (iv) calcitonin and
   (v) vitamin K (although this is still being clinically assessed).

   Although the calcium supplements are less effective than oestrogen, they have fewer side-effects and in this patient it would be advisable to give her calcium.

Discussion

The prevalence of patients with peptic ulcers over the age of 60 years is 15–20%. However, the presentation in elderly patients varies; some may have symptoms similar to younger patients, others have non-specific symptoms including weight loss, vomiting with vague general discomfort. The complication rate is high and perforation can be silent. Half the perforations now occur in those over 70 years of age.

Large giant peptic ulcers may be noted on endoscopy in the elderly and, although they look malignant, they are histologically benign and respond well to medical treatment.

Use of vitamin K in osteoporosis is supported by the following facts:

(i) it reduces calcium excretion in these patient,
(ii) vitamin levels are found to be low in patients with fractured neck of the femur,
(iii) an increase in osteocalcin, a vitamin K-dependent protein, results in increase in bone density and
(iv) osteoporosis of old age, or that associated with steroid therapy, exhibits increased urinary gammacarboxyglutamic acid which reflects increased breakdown of osteocalcin.

Further Reading

James, O., 'Gastrointestinal disorders in the elderly', *International Medicine Gastrointestinal Disorders, Part 3* (1982), **1**, 644–647

'Osteoporosis and its treatment' *Drug and Therapeutics Bulletin* (1984), **22**, 1–4

Gallop, P. M., Lian, J. B. and Hauschka, P. V., 'Carboxylated calcium-binding proteins and vitamin K', *New England Journal of Medicine* (1980) **306**, 1460–1466

Case 51

Answers

1. (i) Prostatic carcinoma,
   (ii) Leucoerythroblastic anaemia,
   (iii) Thoracic radiculopathy or spinal cord compression.
2. Oestrogen with or without nitrogen mustard or orchidectomy or cyproterone blocks the synthesis of androgen and inhibits LH. In addition local irradiation to the dorsal spine may be required for pain relief.
3. The benign treatable conditions which can lead to a leucoerythroblastic blood picture are:
   (i) infection,
   (ii) iron deficiency anaemia,
   (iii) haemorrhage,
   (iv) megaloblastic anaemia,
   (v) coeliac disease,
   (vi) congestive cardiac failure and
   (vi) tuberculosis.

Discussion

Leucoerythroblastic anaemia has been thought to be almost diagnostic of marrow infiltration by tumour tissue but repeated recent reviews highlight the appearance of benign treatable causes of this blood film.

In cases of carcinoma of the prostate where hormonal resistance becomes established because of a predominance of a clone of androgen independent neoplastic cells, chemotherapy may be used to treat the metastatic disease. In those with troublesome bone pain hypophysectomy may be useful.

Further Reading

Creaven, P. J., 'New potential treatment modalities for disseminated prostatic cancer', *Urology Clinics of North America* (1984), **11**, 343–356

Weick, J. K., Hagedorn, A. B. and Linman, J. W., 'Leucoerythroblastosis – diagnostic and prognostic significance', *Mayo Clinic Proceedings* (1974) **49**, 110–114

Case 52

Answers

1. Peaked T waves and prolongation of P wave and QRS complexes. In addition to this, a patient with hyperkalaemia may develop ventricular fibrillation or standstill.
2. Hyperkalaemia was due to amiloride in a patient with impaired renal function. The impaired renal function was confirmed in this patient by the presence of small kidneys on ultrasound.
3. (i) Discontinuation of amiloride,
   (ii) glucose and insulin as well as calcium resonium to correct the hyperkalaemia.

   As a temporary measure to remove the potassium from the blood into the cells, 50 ml (50%) glucose solution with 25 IU soluble insulin should be used. To remove the potassium from the body, calcium resonium should be given, either orally (15 g tds) or by retention enema (30–60 g).

Discussion

Potassium sparing diuretics should be avoided in patients with renal impairment and in those with diabetes mellitus. Serum urea and serum potassium should be checked before starting treatment in the elderly with these conditions.

Further Reading

Bailey, R. R., 'Diuretics and the elderly', *British Medical Journal* (1978), **1**, 1618

Jaffrey, L. and Martin, A., 'Malignant hyperkalaemia after amiloride/hydrochlorothiazide treatment', *Lancet* (1981), **1**, 1272

Case 53

Answers

1. (i) Pseudogout.
   (ii) Infection.
   (iii) Gout.
   (iv) Traumatic effusion.
   The differential diagnosis between these 4 diagnoses can be resolved by tapping the effusion, and sending the fluid for microscopy for cell and crystal examination and also for culture.
2. Chronic polyarticular gout.
3. In view of the daughter-in-law's objection the patient should be assessed at home by an occupational therapist, preferably in the presence of the daughter-in-law to demonstrate the patient's capabilities. If the home visit is a success then it will be possible to discharge her home with appropriate support from the community; if not, the patient would have appreciated it and, hopefully, this would have made her more amenable to accepting other permanent placement such as Part III accommodation. If in this situation however, the patient still insists on going home we have no option but to let her go with close supervision particularly from the social services in case she

deteriorates and reaches a stage where she requires to go into a home as an emergency.

Discussion

Gout not only presents with intermittent acute arthritis of one joint but also with chronic polyarticular involvement. The latter presentation tends to occur in women who are on diuretic therapy. The chronic arthritis may be misdiagnosed since, in some cases, it may present with symmetrical joint involvement.

Treatment of the condition is with use of allopurinol under the cover of a non-steroidal anti-inflammatory agent. An acute episode should be treated with anti-inflammatory agents such as azapropazone or indomethacin or colchicine.

Further Reading

Schousboe, J. T., Davey, K., Gilchrist, N. L. and Sainsbury, R., 'Chronic polyarticular gout in the elderly – a report of six cases', *Age and Ageing* (1986), **15**, 8–16

Case 54

Answers

1. (i) Brainstem cerebrovascular accident.
   (ii) Diabetes mellitus.
   (iii) Secondary erythrocytosis due to chronic obstructive airways disease.
   (iv) Atrial fibrillation.
2. (i) Secondary erythrocytosis.
   (ii) Embolism secondary to atrial fibrillation.
   (iii) Probable hypotensive episode secondary to myocardial ischaemia.
3. (i) Nursing care to prevent pressure scores, contractures and loss of muscle.
   (ii) Physiotherapy.
   (iii) Diet for diabetes mellitis.

(iv) Cessation of diuretic therapy to lower packed cell volume.
(v) Venesection to improve viscosity (N.B. Blood volume must be maintained by infusing dextran or dextrose).

Discussion

Atrial fibrillation is a well-known and proven risk factor for embolic disease. However, anticoagulation although indicated, should not be given before cerebral haemorrhage has been excluded by CT scan. In this patient, anticoagulant therapy was not given because of his past history of hypertension.

There are many correctable risk factors that lead to recurrent strokes and these include hypertension, diabetes mellitus, hyperlipidaemia, atherosclerotic disease of aorto-cervical and intracranial arteries, arteriosclerotic heart disease, polycythaemia, smoking and obesity.

For the atherosclerotic disease (affecting carotid territories) presenting with TIAs aspirin has been shown to be beneficial by some studies in men. On theoretical grounds, a small dose should be used since it has been shown that higher doses of aspirin (i.e. >80 mg/day) may inhibit vascular production of the natural anti-platelet and vasodilator substance, prostacyclin. Extracranial to intracranial bypass surgery has been tried but has not been shown to produce any benefit.

There is no doubt that hypertension is an important risk factor for stroke in the older person. Treatment has been shown by the recent report of European Working Party in hypertension (1985) to lead to significant reduction in both cardiac and cerebrovascular events. However, all anti-hypertensive therapies have side-effects and these are particularly common in the elderly.

Further Reading

Gavras, H. and Gavras, I., 'Risk of stroke in the hypertensive elderly patient', *Geriatric Medicine Today* (1985), **4**, 72–75
Frackowiak, R., 'Comment – the use of anti-platelet drugs in transient ischaemic attacks and stroke', *Current Medical*

Literature Neurology The Royal Society of Medicine (1984), 1, 4–7

Amery, A. *et al.*, 'Mortality and morbidity results from the European Working party on high blood pressure in the elderly trial', *Lancet* (1985), 1, 1349–1354

Case 55

Answers

1. (i) Tetraparesis secondary to Paget's disease, or metastases from prostatic carcinoma, or both.
   (ii) Non-insulin dependent diabetes mellitus.
   (iii) Iron deficiency anaemia.
   (iv) Hypophosphataemic osteomalacia.
2. The hypophosphataemia in this patient is the result of prostatic carcinoma. Profound hypophosphataemia may be caused by:
   (i) alcohol withdrawal,
   (ii) diabetes mellitus,
   (iii) the binding of phosphate by aluminium hydroxide and magnesium hydroxide,
   (iv) during the recovery phase from severe burns,
   (v) hyperalimentation and
   (vi) severe respiratory alkalosis.
3. The treatment this patient received was:
   (i) dietary advice for non-insulin dependent diabetes mellitus,
   (ii) replacement supplements for iron deficiency,
   (iii) oestrogen therapy (stilboestrol 1 mg/day) for carcinoma of the prostate,
   (iv) 1 α-hydroxy vitamin D (1 μg bd) for the hypophosphataemic osteomalacia and
   (v) physiotherapy.
4. The patient will be given a full explanation about the cause of his symptoms, the treatment he requires and the likely side-effects of the drugs in order to improve compliance. The actual term 'cancer' will be used only if the patient brings it out in discussion.

Discussion

Hypophosphataemic osteomalacia associated with carcinoma of the prostate is common in the elderly. The characteristic features are a low renal phosphate threshold concentration, a normal parathyroid hormone level, normal 25-hydroxy D3 but low 1, 25 dihydroxy D3. The symptoms in these patients, which include not only muscle weakness but pain, improve with alfacalcidol treatment together with specific therapy for carcinoma of the prostate.

Further Reading

Murphy, P., Wright, G. and Rai, G. S., 'Hypophosphataemic osteomalacia associated with prostatic carcinoma', *British Medical Journal* (1985) **290**, 194

Knochel, J. P., 'The pathophysiology and clinical characteristics of severe hypophosphataemia', *Archives of Internal Medicine* (1977), **137**, 203–219

Case 56

Answers

1. The most likely cause is pseudomembraneous colitis caused by the antibiotic prescribed 3 weeks earlier for bronchopneumonia. The diagnosis can be confirmed by rectal biopsy, detection of *Clostridium difficile* toxin or by positive culture for *Clostridium difficile* from faeces.
2. Treatment consists of rehydration and use of vancomycin (125 mg qds) or metronidazole. Prognosis is poor in the elderly, with the mortality varying from 27–70%.
3. The future plan will depend upon:
   (i) the level of independence achieved after the treatment and rehabilitation and
   (ii) on the patient's own wishes.

   If the patient wishes to return home then a home visit should be performed in view of the 2 recent admissions to hospital over a short interval.

Discussion

Antibiotic-associated colitis or pseudomembranous colitis is due to proliferation of *Clostridium difficile* in the colon. This occurs when the normal flora has been suppressed by an antibiotic. Many antibiotics produce this iatrogenic illness. The patient usually presents with diarrhoea without bleeding. Other features that may be present include fever, low albumin and leucocytosis.

Any elderly patient presenting with diarrhoea should be investigated to find a cause which not only includes pseudomembranous colitis, but overflow diarrhoea associated with impaction, infective diarrhoea, diverticular disease of colon, carcinoma of large bowel, Crohn's disease, ulcerative colitis, ischaemic colitis and malabsorption.

Further Reading

Roddis, M. J. 'Antibiotic associated colitis', *Age and Ageing* (1978), **7**, 182–188

Case 57

Answers

1. Biventricular failure possible secondary to:
   (i) ischaemic heart disease,
   (ii) subacute bacterial endocarditis,
   (iii) occult valvular disease and
   (iv) senile cardiac amyloidosis.
2. (i) Blood cultures (three),
   (ii) echocardiogram.
3. Initial treatment should be with the use of diuretics (i.e. frusemide with amiloride). If this has a limited effect addition of digoxin or drugs which reduce preload or 'after load' should be considered (e.g. prazosin, captopril, enalapril).

Discussion

The presence of senile cardiac amyloidosis rises with age. However, only when the deposition is of grade II–IV does it lead to cardiac abnormalities varying from atrial fibrillation to heart failure. Classically, the cardiac failure occurs without chest pain or without evidence of valvular disease. On examination, these patients may have a gallop rhythm or signs of pericardial tamponade. On ECG testing the complexes are of low voltage and there are T-wave changes. Currently the diagnosis can only be made at post mortem as rectal biopsy which is useful in detecting secondary amyloid tends to be negative in these patients.

In ischaemic heart disease, acute myocardial infarction may present either with chest pain or without chest pain but with an acute confusional state, syncopal attacks, hemiplegia, vomiting, intense weakness or even renal failure without pain in the chest.

Reducing excessive preload of the failing heart improves symptoms due to congestion. The reduction in preload can be achieved by salt restriction, diuretics and with the use of venous vasodilators such as isosorbide dinitrate. A decrease in afterload (which is determined by arterial impedence and which is in turn determined by systemic resistance) allows the cardiac output to increase. In intractable heart failure, drugs which reduce preload or afterload or both can be tried. It is preferable to use drugs which reduce both preload and afterload (i.e. have an arterial dilating action as well as a venous pooling effect (e.g. captopril or enalapril).

Further Reading

Hodkinson, H. M. and Pomerance, A., 'The clinical significance of senile cardiac amyloidosis. Prospective clinico-pathological study', *Quarterly Journal of Medicine (NS)* (1977), **XLVI,** 381–387

Buja, M. L., Khoi, N. B. A. and Roberts, W. C., 'Clinically significant cardiac amyloidosis. Clinico-pathologic finding in 15 patients', *American Journal of Cardiology* (1970), **26,** 394–408

Little, R. C. and Little, W. C., 'Cardiac preload, afterload and heart failure', *Archives of Internal Medicine* (1982), **142,** 819–822

Macdonald, J. B., 'Presentation of acute myocardial infarction in the elderly – a review', *Age and Ageing* (1984), **13**, 196–200

Case 58

Answers

1. The main problems in this patient were the result of polypharmacy. He had features of digoxin toxicity and dehydration. The former was confirmed by the digoxin level of 6.09 nmol/l.
2. (i) Stop the digoxin and diuretic therapy. In view of the valvular disease and atrial fibrillation, he may again require these drugs once the toxic-effects have resolved.
   (ii) Stop the methyldopa and observe the blood pressure. It is possible he may not require this.
3. This patient probably does not require the steroids. Although the activity of polymyalgia rheumatica can go on for many years, it is usually a self-limiting disease; thus it is advisable to curtail administration of steroids after 1 to 2 years of therapy. If the patient's symptoms return, the steroids can be recommenced.

Discussion

Digitalis toxicity increases with advancing age of patients and with deteriorating renal function. A toxic reaction is more likely to occur in patients with myocardial damage, during hypoxia or hypokalaemia. However, this does not mean that digoxin is contra-indicated in the elderly. It is still used and is the drug of choice in supraventricular arrhythmia such as atrial fibrillation and in selected patients with heart failure.

Polypharmacy is hazardous as illustrated in this case. Not only can it lead to drug interaction but adverse effects and poor compliance. Interactions are especially liable to occur with anticoagulants, antidepressants, anticonvulsants, cardioglycosides, hypoglycaemic agents and antihypertensive agents.

Further Reading

'Editorial: digitalis update', *Archives of Internal Medicine* (1981) **141**, 17–18

'Editorial: digitalis in cardiac failure' *Archives of Internal Medicine* (1981), **141**, 18–19

Case 59

Answers

1. Bullous eruptions can be a feature of pemphigoid, pemphigus, erythema multiforme, contact dermatitis, herpes simplex, drug reactions or trauma.
2. The diagnosis can be confirmed by skin biopsy, and by demonstration of antibodies which in pemphigoid are against the basement membrane.
3. Oral steroids. Starting doses should be 40–60 mg per day, but this should be tapered according to response.
4. Causes of eosinophilia are:
   (i) allergic conditions (e.g. asthma and urticaria),
   (ii) skin conditions (e.g. pemphigoid, pemphigus eczema, mycosis and fungoides),
   (iii) parasitic infestations (e.g. trichiniasis),
   (iv) haematological conditions (e.g. polycythaemia, myelocytic leukaemia and Hodgkin's disease),
   (v) following drug usage (e.g. nitrofurantoin, paraminosalicylic acid, sulphonamide or penicillin), and
   (vi) miscellaneous conditions (e.g. rheumatoid arthritis, sarcoidosis, following splenectomy, irradiation and malignancy).

Discussion

Pemphigoid is a relatively benign bullous condition of the elderly. It responds to steroids and may eventually 'burn itself out'. It may be confused with pemphigus but differentiating features are:

(i) blisters are thin in pemphigus,
(ii) on histology the blisters show acantholysis and antibodies are found to be against epidermal cells rather than the basement membrane,
(iii) mucous membranes are more frequently involved in pemphigus than pemphigoid.
(iv) pemphigus is a serious condition and can lead to death if left untreated.

Case 60

Answers

1. Haematoma with femoral nerve compression.
2. Whole blood clotting studies were performed to see if the patient had been over-anticoagulated; the treatment consisted of infusion of fresh frozen plasma and blood. Surgical drainage of the haematoma in this patient was not considered because symptoms improved with medical treatment.

Discussion

Elderly women are more prone to bleeding episodes when treated with heparin. This may be related to reduced protein binding in the sick elderly patient who tends to have low albumin levels. In most cases the complication of haemorrhage can be overcome by controlling the dosage according to whole blood clotting time.

However, as this case demonstrates, haemorrhage can occur even with close monitoring. Warfarin, like heparin, can also lead to bleeding in the elderly as they seem to be more sensitive to this drug than younger patients. This does not mean that the elderly should not be given anticoagulants. Those whose condition warrants anticoagulation (i.e. those with extensive deep vein thrombosis, pulmonary embolism, systemic embolism or those with rheumatic heart disease) should be given it; however, patients need to be monitored closely, particularly in relation to the administration of other drugs.

Further Reading

Jick, H., Slone, D., Borda, I. T. and Shapiro, S., 'Efficiency and toxicity of heparin in relation to age and sex', *New England Journal of Medicine* (1968), **279,** 284–286

O'Malley, K., Stevenson, I. H., Ward, C. A. Wood, A. J. J. and Crooks, J., 'Determinants of anticoagulant control in patients receiving warfarin', *British Journal of Clinical Pharmacology* (1977) **4,** 309–314

Normal Laboratory Values which are Different in the Elderly

Haematological Indices

Haemoglobin (Men): 11.8–16.8 g/dl
Haemoglobin (Women): 11.1–15.5 g/dl
MCV: 82–96 fl
HCT (Men): 42–54%
HCT (Women): 36–48%
WCC: 3.1–8.9 × 10^9/l
Serum iron: 8.8–30.3 μmol/l
TIBC: 38.3–87.0 μmol/l

Biochemical Indices

Albumin: 33–49 g/l
Alkaline phosphatase: 30–115 IU/l
Calcium (Men): 2.19–2.60 mmol/l
Calcium (Women): 2.18–2.68 mmol/l
Caeruloplasmin: 0.213–0.507 g/l
Copper: 13.06–30.62 μmol/l
Creatinine: 52–159 μmol/l
Globulin: 33–49 g/l
Potassium: 3.5–5.2 mmol/l
Phosphate (Men): 0.66–1.27 mmol/l
Phosphate (Women): 0.94–1.56 mmol/l
Urate (Men): 0.19–0.31 mmol/l
Urate (Women): 0.13–0.46 mmol/l
Zinc: 8.54–17.02 μmol/l

Further Reading

Hodkinson, M., 'Biochemical changes in old age', *Medicine International* (1983), **1** (36), 1701–1703

Coodley, E., Ofstein, M., Coodley, G. and Rick, J., 'Correlation of laboratory values with ageing', *Geriatric Medicine Today* (1986), **5**, 29–39

Hale, W. E., Stewart, R. B. and Marks, R. G., 'Haematological and biochemical laboratory values in an ambulatory elderly population: an analysis of the effects of age, sex and drugs', *Age and Ageing* (1983), **12**, 275–284

Index